AF869178

THE GRAND FORKS RIVER OF PROTECTION

A Long Essay on the Work, Persistence, and Quiet Triumph of

Dr. Nicholas VC Ralston and the Selenium-Mercury Paradigm

By Joe Cozart

on behalf of GMJoe™ Consulting

DEDICATION

For the mothers who were told the wrong story,

for the children who deserved a truer one,

and for the scientist who never stopped showing up

on behalf of both.

EPIGRAPH

“Clarity is not what arrives first.

Clarity is what remains after everything else dissolves.”

ANTEROOM

This work began in the quiet corridors of a northern campus, where the winters are long and the truth moves slowly. It emerged not from certainty, but from a scientist's refusal to accept a story that never aligned with the evidence. What follows is not a biography, nor a scientific treatise, nor a policy argument. It is literary nonfiction, the record of a decades-long correction—one that traveled from laboratory benches to global symposiums, from coastal clinics to international policy rooms, from lonely whiteboards to the inherited knowledge of a new generation. It is the story of how a single insight became a current that reshaped the world, quietly, steadily, inevitably.

PREFACE

Every field has its moment of convergence—the instant when resistance dissolves, the paradigm settles, and what once required defense becomes simply the way things are understood. The selenium-mercury interaction model reached that moment not through force, but through endurance. This essay traces the arc of that endurance: the early hesitations, the lonely years, the global recalibration, and the inherence that followed. It is a long-form exploration in which science becomes narrative and clarity becomes time. Nothing here is exaggerated; the quiet revolutions never are.

ACKNOWLEDGMENT OF CONTEXT

This essay exists because of two forces:

the uncompromising discipline of scientific truth,

and the rare individual who refused to let that truth be buried by fear.

The work of Dr. Nicholas VC Ralston spans more than two decades and intersects biochemistry, maternal health, international policy, and the politics of scientific messaging. His persistence corrected a generation of misunderstanding. This essay stands not as a monument, but as a record—an account of what clarity looks like when carried through every season of resistance.

TABLE OF CONTENTS

COPYRIGHT PAGE

The Grand Forks River of Protection

© 2025 by Joe Cozart. All rights reserved.

No part of this book may be reproduced or transmitted in any form or by any means, electronic or mechanical, including photocopying or recording, without prior written permission from the publisher.

GMJoe™ Consulting

Grand Forks, North Dakota

GMJoe™ is a trademark of Joe Cozart. © 2025 All rights reserved.

ISBN: 978-1-970547-07-8

Printed in the United States of America.

There are truths that enter the world without ceremony, so small at first that their significance is indistinguishable from inconvenience. They arrive quietly, like the faint clicking of a distant instrument in a laboratory after midnight, or the way a winter wind leans against the old stone of a northern university building before settling into its long exhale. What follows is never a revelation. It is endurance. And it was into this endurance that a scientist in Grand Forks found himself drawn, not out of design or destiny, but because he noticed something the rest of the field had learned to overlook.

It began, as most scientific heresies do, with an imbalance. The prevailing doctrine — repeated in advisories, in policy briefs, in conversations between physicians and anxious expectant mothers — insisted that the danger lay in the fish themselves, that the sea had become treacherous, that mercury was the silent adversary gathering in the muscle of ocean species and waiting to sabotage fetal development. This idea was easy to teach, easy to warn against, easy to fear. Entire careers had been built on its repetition. It had the advantage of simplicity, and institutions cling to simplicity the way a cold building clings to its last stored heat in January.

Yet in the quiet arithmetic of molecular life, simplicity is often the first casualty. And it was in this arithmetic — in the biochemical companionship of selenium and mercury — that the scientist began to see a different architecture forming, one that did not conform to what the committees and conferences were prepared to acknowledge. The body did not treat mercury as an isolated force. It treated it as an interruption. And what mattered most was not the presence of mercury, but the availability of selenium to continue its indispensable work. There was, in other words, a ratio.

A relationship. A balance that governed whether harm could occur at all.

Most people would have noted the finding, published the paper, and returned to the safer territories of consensus. But he saw something else inside the data — a kind of structural mercy built into ocean life, a principle that had gone unrecognized because fear had drawn too much attention to the wrong element. Fish did not threaten the fetus. They protected it, so long as their selenium outpaced their mercury. The very species that had been condemned in public advisories were, by biochemical design, among the most reliable guardians of early brain development.

It was an insight too elegant to be quickly accepted. Institutions distrust elegance. Committees distrust correction. And the scientific world, like all worlds, had learned to prefer the familiar superstition over the unfamiliar truth. Yet he kept returning to it — year after year, winter after winter — walking the same corridors at the university long after the building had emptied, refining the measurements, re-examining the patterns, testing whether the truth would fracture under pressure. It did not. The deeper he went, the clearer the architecture became.

But clarity is not the same as acceptance. And so the scientist found himself in the familiar position of anyone who recognizes a truth before its era is ready to carry it: he had to bear the burden of repetition. To advisory boards. To public health committees. To rooms full of experts who nodded politely, then returned to the doctrine that had preceded him. The world had rehearsed its fear for too many years to surrender it easily. Mercury had become the villain, and fish the accomplice, and no amount of biochemical proportion could persuade them otherwise.

Still, he continued. Not out of defiance, but out of duty to the developing brain — that delicate, unfolding sovereignty that required nutrients so essential that nature had devised a molecular shield to protect them. He understood what the committees did not: that the true danger was not the presence of mercury in fish, but the absence of fish in the diets of those who needed their protection most. To remove fish out of fear was to remove the very defense that guarded the fetus from harm.

And so the lights stayed on late in Grand Forks. The work continued in winters long enough to outlast optimism, in seasons where only the stubborn remain. There was no glory in it. No applause. Only the quiet conviction that a generation was being misled by a superstition its own scientists had built, and that someone had to untangle the error before it hardened into permanence.

He did not set out to become a corrective force in the world — no one ever does — yet there was something in the nature of the work that refused to leave him untouched. Once a person sees the architecture behind an illusion, it becomes impossible to unsee it. And so the scientist found himself living inside a paradox: the world believed the sea was dangerous, while he was discovering — molecule by molecule, enzyme by enzyme — that the real danger was the hunger created by fear itself.

For decades, public guidance had taught expectant mothers to avoid the very foods that had once nourished entire civilizations through gestation. Warnings spread with the efficiency of rumor, and as decades passed, the caution hardened into doctrine. Physicians repeated it. Agencies codified it. Mothers internalized it. An entire generation learned to distrust its own ancestry. And in the northern plains, where winters rarely forgive hesitation, the man who understood the truth watched as the fear became policy, and policy became culture.

Yet science does not bend toward culture. Science bends toward proportion.

And the proportions were unmistakable.

The fetus needed long-chain omega-3s with a desperation that could not be spoken aloud — not in newspapers, not in pamphlets, not in the careful language of advisory boards. The developing brain is not metaphor; it is architecture in motion. It requires a constant flow of the raw materials that form synapses, insulate neurons, and guide the early choreography of cognition. Without these materials, development falters. With them, it flourishes. And in the ocean's long memory, fish had evolved the biochemical shield — selenium — that prevented mercury from interrupting that choreography.

But the world had grown too enamored with its own alarm to hear this.

Over the years, the scientist learned to recognize the look: the polite pause in a conference room; the tightening around the eyes of a committee member; the subtle bracing of an agency representative who knew the political cost of revising a public warning. They were not hostile. They were tethered. Bound by the momentum of past statements, past studies, past fears. To change course was to admit they had misinterpreted a threat. Bureaucracies do not metabolize humility easily.

And so he spoke the truth in smaller rooms, to smaller audiences, knowing that revolutions in public health rarely begin with declarations. They begin with persistence. He refined the data. He repeated the findings. He traveled to speak with those willing to listen, and those unwilling to hear. He answered questions from people who assumed the old narrative was the only narrative. He watched as well-intentioned professionals repeated warnings they had inherited rather than examined.

In the isolation of the upper Midwest, where the wind seems to strip everything down to its barest form, he practiced a kind of scientific patience that borders on devotion. While others built careers around crises, he built a career around correction. While others spoke of danger, he spoke of balance. While others measured risk, he measured proportion. And though he carried no banner and led no movement, his work was becoming, slowly and quietly, a kind of resistance — a stand against a misunderstanding that had lasted too long and cost too much.

He understood something the agencies did not:

that a fear repeated often enough becomes indistinguishable from truth,

and a truth repeated too softly becomes indistinguishable from silence.

This was the burden he carried.

Not the data.

Not the science.

The silence.

For silence can be heavier than error, far heavier than the mercury others feared. It can suffocate the very knowledge designed to protect the vulnerable. And so he resolved, in his unadorned way, to keep speaking until the silence broke — even if it took the rest of his life.

Winter after winter, he returned to the lab, the office, the long unlit hallways of the university where only custodial lights remained. Papers stacked. Data refined. Ratios recalculated. Presentations rewritten. Letters answered. Entire evenings spent testing whether the truth could withstand one more challenge, one more hostile interpretation, one more institutional reluctance.

And it always did.

Because the truth was not complicated. Only the courage to revise the doctrine was.

The ratio held.

It held through scrutiny.

It held through criticism.

It held through review.

It held through the inertia of institutions determined to protect their earlier conclusions rather than the children those conclusions were intended to serve.

And every time it held, he understood the same thing:

He was not correcting a scientific misunderstanding.

He was correcting a generational one.

There are moments in a scientist's life when the work stops being an exercise in inquiry and becomes something closer to an obligation — not imposed by institutions or expectations, but by the quiet recognition that no one else will carry what must be carried. Somewhere in the long stretch of years, without any ceremony or declaration, he understood that his task was no longer to persuade the scientific world. It was to protect the unborn from the consequences of its confusion.

He never said this aloud. Men like him rarely do. But there was a shift, a barely perceptible turning of the inner compass, when he realized he was no longer arguing a point of biochemistry. He was holding a line. A line between fear and fact. Between old assumptions and the molecular truth that contradicted them. Between a world that thought it understood the sea and a sea that had been misunderstood for generations.

Most people think scientific progress happens through breakthroughs — single moments of clarity that reorder everything that came before. But his world was one of accretion: small studies, incremental refinements, meticulous recalculations that together formed a bulwark against the error that dominated public conversation. He became fluent in the long patience of molecular correction, where each experiment was less an act of discovery and more an act of confirmation: the ratio still held. The relationship between selenium and mercury was not fragile. It was resilient, repeating itself across species, across ecosystems, across years of scrutiny.

The world could shift its fears, but the molecules did not.

And yet the institutions responsible for shaping public guidance behaved as though the molecules were merely suggestions. Warnings remained unchanged. Advisories remained anchored to outdated interpretations. Mercury retained its place as the central villain, and fish — the very reservoirs of protection — remained cast in the role of accomplice. This was not deception; it was inertia. Bureaucratic systems have a tendency to crystallize around the earliest story they tell, even after the story has been disproven.

He learned to navigate these systems with the understanding of a man who had become more archaeologist than advocate. Each policy document was a dig through layers of institutional sediment, uncovering outdated assumptions buried beneath the polite language of public health. He was patient with the individuals — scientists, policymakers, physicians — because he knew the struggle was not against people, but against the momentum of their predecessors.

Still, there were nights when even patience could not disguise the cost. Nights when the exhaustion crept in, not from the work itself, but from the knowledge that the delay had consequences. Every year the warnings went uncorrected was another year of pregnancies guided away from the foods designed by evolutionary necessity to nourish the brain. Every year the committees postponed recalibration was another year of children born without the full benefit of what the sea had provided since the earliest memory of human nutrition.

In the long quiet of the northern plains, these thoughts gathered with the same stillness as snow in the hours before dawn. There was an acute loneliness in knowing the truth and watching it move so slowly through the world. Yet he never once considered leaving the field. Working elsewhere would have changed nothing. The misunderstanding would continue without him, calcifying into permanence.

So he stayed.

And the university around him — long winters, long hallways, long silences — became less a workplace and more a kind of observatory. A place from which he watched the world rehearse its fear with such conviction that even well-meaning professionals became unwitting participants in a slow-moving harm. He learned to distinguish between the noise of public discourse and the deeper signal of molecular reality. One could be deafening. The other was steady.

In this steadiness, he found a form of resolve.

Not the defiance of a crusader, but the tenacity of a man who knows that the world eventually returns to proportion, even if it must be dragged back molecule by molecule. He did not think of himself as carrying a generational burden, though he was. He thought only of the next study, the next presentation, the next meeting where he would sit before yet another committee attempting to convince them that the ocean was not guilty of the crimes they had assigned to it.

And each time he spoke — calmly, precisely, without flourish — he was not offering an argument. He was offering a return to truth.

Because in the end, the science was simple:

If selenium exceeds mercury, the child is safe.

Everything else was noise.

Everything else was the echo of old fear.

There is a kind of fatigue that never announces itself outright — it gathers gradually, like frost along the edges of a windowpane, subtle enough to ignore until the room itself begins to feel colder. He lived with this fatigue for years. It was not the weariness of labor; the experiments, the analysis, the long hours at the university were not what weighed on him. It was the knowledge that the distance between truth and adoption could span entire generations, and that during that span, harm could persist simply because no one wished to revise an inherited warning.

It is difficult for people to admit they were misled by good intentions. Harder still for institutions. And so he learned to speak into rooms where he knew, beforehand, that his words would fall into the soft cushion of polite dismissal. Committees would nod. Specialists would acknowledge his expertise. Advisors would agree, in principle, that his data were compelling. But when the meeting ended, they returned to the language that preceded him. Not out of malice, but habit. Fear had a longer half-life than the evidence.

He came to understand that he was not presenting information — he was asking the world to change its mind. And the world, particularly the part governed by risk-averse agencies, does not change its mind because a single scientist has produced the correct ratio.

Still, he persisted.

He persisted because the ratio was not merely scientific. It was moral. It spoke to a deeper responsibility: the obligation to protect the developing brain not just from toxins, but from the consequences of collective misunderstanding. The fetus is the most vulnerable expression of human potential, unable to defend itself, dependent on the nourishment selected on its behalf. To deprive it of the very nutrients designed by nature to orchestrate its formation — out of an excess of precaution rooted in an error — was not a small matter. It was a quiet injury, repeated millions of times with official approval.

This was the part he never expressed in public. Scientists are trained to speak in cautious language, to avoid moral indictment. But the moral dimension lived beneath the work, the way a river runs beneath winter ice — invisible but forceful. When he explained the selenium-mercury relationship, he chose his words carefully. He never spoke of harm, only of possibility. He never accused, only clarified. It was not his style to tell anyone they were wrong. He preferred to show why the truth was simpler than the story that had replaced it.

Yet he was not immune to frustration. There were days when he watched a public health pamphlet circulate, offering warnings untouched by the research he had presented for years, and he felt a wave of quiet disbelief. The pamphlet looked authoritative. It wore the insignias of legitimacy. It bore the weight of federal language. And yet its guidance, delivered with the confidence of settled knowledge, would have been corrected decades earlier if institutions moved at the speed of evidence rather than the pace of bureaucracy.

Still, he did not yield to cynicism. Cynicism was an indulgence he could not afford. The work demanded clarity, not bitterness. He could not allow himself to resent the institutions he hoped to change. He could not afford to alienate the very people whose minds he needed to reach. And so he developed an unusual form of scientific composure: an almost monastic patience, unshakeable, steady, anchored not in personality but in fidelity to proportion.

He did not win converts quickly. Science rarely changes through persuasion alone. It changes through persistence that outlasts resistance. And so he continued — repeating the same truths in conference halls and small offices, in policy discussions and research meetings, in conversations with health professionals who had never once questioned the origin of their warnings.

Sometimes he wondered whether the message would only be accepted when the next generation of scientists took over — a generation unburdened by the old doctrine, willing to see the relationship between selenium and mercury without the residue of inherited fear. He did not resent this possibility. He had long ago accepted that he might not be the one to witness the full correction. The work was not for his recognition. It was for the unborn who would one day benefit from guidance grounded in biological accuracy rather than cultural memory.

What he did witness, over time, was a slow shift — the faintest cracks in the old narrative. A paper published that cited his findings. A conference discussion that cautiously entertained his implications. A policymaker asking, privately, for clarification. These were not victories, but signals. The first signs that the architecture of misinformation, so firmly built, was beginning to soften.

It was enough.

Because he knew the truth possessed a structural integrity the error lacked. The error needed constant reinforcement — pamphlets, advisories, warnings, campaigns. The truth needed none. It simply existed, waiting to be recognized. And he trusted the world, eventually, to rediscover its proportions.

For in the end, all ratios seek equilibrium.

And this one — selenium to mercury — had been waiting for decades to reclaim its rightful place in the guidance given to those whose decisions shape the earliest moments of human life.

There were mornings in Grand Forks when the world seemed to pause before revealing itself — when the sun rose reluctantly over the flat horizon, washing the campus in a muted, pearlescent light that made the laboratories look almost ceremonial. He often arrived before the first of the undergraduates filtered through the doors. The silence felt different at that hour: not empty, but expectant, like the stillness before an orchestra begins to tune. These early hours had become his private territory, the time when the noise of public misunderstanding had not yet seeped into the day.

The long hallways of the university had a way of reminding him that his work belonged to a timeline larger than his own. Institutions endure. Buildings outlast their occupants. The generations who walked these corridors before him had fought their own battles against error, superstition, and institutional inertia. Some had succeeded. Some had been forgotten. He understood he was not the first to try to correct a public misconception, nor would he be the last. But he also understood that the magnitude of a misconception is not measured by its visibility, but by the quiet damage it inflicts over time.

Most people think harm must be immediate to be real. But the harm he saw — the harm that animated every late night, every recalculated dataset — was cumulative. It was the harm of absence rather than presence. The harm of deprivation rather than exposure. The harm of a nutrient withheld not out of malice, but out of caution rooted in an outdated belief.

This, he knew, was the most difficult kind of harm to correct: the harm born from good intentions.

Mothers avoided fish because they loved their children. Doctors made the recommendation because they wished to protect. Agencies issued warnings because they imagined they were preventing catastrophe. The entire misunderstanding was built atop the most sympathetic motives — and that, paradoxically, made it harder to unwind. Fear justified as responsibility becomes almost religious in its persistence.

He saw this at conferences, especially those focused on maternal health. The rooms were always full — physicians, researchers, public health officials, nutritionists — people who had devoted their lives to protecting vulnerable populations. They listened closely, asked thoughtful questions, took notes. But when the conversation shifted back to recommendations, the room reverted to its familiar script. Avoid high-mercury fish. Be cautious. Err on the side of safety. They could not see that what they called safety was, at the molecular level, the opposite.

Sometimes, after leaving such meetings, he would walk the length of the campus rather than return immediately to his office. Walking seemed to clear the residue of frustration. The wind — relentless, disciplined — served as a reminder that the world did not bend easily to one man's insistence. It had its own tempo. Its own resistance. The wind did not care whether he succeeded. It did not care what institutions feared. It moved with indifference, carving the plains into their quiet shapes.

In that indifference, he found an odd comfort.

Because his work was not personal. He was not trying to win a debate or prove himself right. He was trying to prevent a misunderstanding from becoming permanent — trying to make sure that the developing brain, so exquisitely vulnerable, received the full protection nature had intended. The ocean had done its part. The molecules had done theirs. Only the message had gone astray.

And messages, however entrenched, could be corrected.

He suspected the real obstacle was not the complexity of his findings but the simplicity of them. People expect danger to be direct, not relational. They expect toxins to be harmful on their own, not only in the absence of a protective counterpart. They expect the world to be governed by isolated forces, not by ratios. Ratios confound fear. They require context, proportion, and patience — qualities not easily translated into public advisories.

But he had never been drawn to the dramatic or the sensational. His temperament aligned more closely with the quiet mechanics of biology: enzymes working without fanfare, molecules binding without declaration, systems protecting without needing acknowledgment. Perhaps that was why he remained so steady through the years — the work itself modeled the behavior required to sustain it.

He continued because the ratio continued.

He endured because the truth endured.

He persisted because the unborn could not.

There were, however, moments — fleeting but unmistakable — when he sensed a shift. A young researcher citing his work without agenda. A clinician reconsidering long-held assumptions. A policy advisor reaching out with a question that suggested true reconsideration rather than bureaucratic ritual. These small signals mattered. They meant the silence was breaking, not loudly, not suddenly, but in the way ice thins beneath the first warmth of spring: quietly, inevitably, almost imperceptibly.

And he understood then that he was not laboring in futility. He was planting a correction that the next generation might harvest. He did not need to see the full transformation. He only needed to ensure that the misunderstanding could no longer claim inevitability.

The truth had entered the world.

It would take time, but it would stay.

There is a particular kind of loneliness reserved for those who see what others have not yet learned to recognize. It is not the loneliness of isolation, nor the loneliness of rejection, but something quieter — a solitude that forms when a person carries knowledge that the world is not prepared to integrate. He lived within that solitude for years without announcing it, without lamenting it, without ever allowing it to harden into bitterness. It became, in time, simply the atmosphere in which the work occurred.

What sustained him was not affirmation, nor the hope of rapid adoption, but the unmistakable clarity of the molecular relationship itself. Selenium and mercury — bound in a rivalry so ancient it predated science, policy, and human interpretation altogether — did not argue. They simply behaved. And the predictability of their behavior offered him a kind of companionship. While committees hesitated and agencies retreated to caution, the molecules remained steadfast, reenacting their proportional logic in every species he examined.

This was the part of the story that most people misunderstood: he was not guessing. He was not theorizing in the abstract. He was observing a pattern that repeated with the reliability of a natural law. The fish of the open ocean carried more selenium than mercury, and therefore they posed no threat to the fetus. The fish that lacked this advantage were few, and easily identified. The protective architecture was already there — nature had built it — but fear had obscured it behind a veil of exaggerated caution.

He sometimes wondered how much of human suffering came from this basic condition — the tendency to fear what is visible rather than what is consequential. Mercury had a name; selenium had a function. One evoked alarm; the other was quietly essential. And because fear moves faster than understanding, the warnings proliferated long before the protective ratio was understood. Once established, the warnings became self-perpetuating, reinforced by repetition rather than accuracy.

He spent years trying to explain that the danger did not lie in the presence of mercury but in the absence of selenium. This inversion — so simple, so biologically obvious to him — remained elusive for those who had internalized the old doctrine. Most people are not trained to think in counterbalances. They think in binaries: harmful or safe, toxic or nutritious, dangerous or benign. But biology is seldom binary. It is relational, interdependent, contextual. He had learned this early in his career, long before the selenium-mercury insight took shape.

That early discipline — the study of enzymes, the intricate dance of nutrients within the body — prepared him for the ratio long before he could articulate it. He knew the body was not governed by isolated forces. It was a network of checks, safeguards, redundancies. It had evolved not only to survive threats, but to outmaneuver them. Selenium was one such outmaneuver: a micronutrient that neutralized mercury's interference with the brain's most delicate processes.

He took comfort in knowing that the body understood what the guidelines did not.

In time, he learned to see the world as a kind of parallel structure to the systems he studied. Policy, like metabolism, had its own bottlenecks. Institutions, like enzymes, had their own activation thresholds. Public opinion behaved like a refractory element — resistant to change until conditions shifted just enough to permit recalibration. And just as the body required a minimum concentration of selenium to protect the brain, the world required a minimum concentration of truth before it could protect itself from error.

He knew he was contributing to that concentration slowly, steadily, molecule by molecule, meeting by meeting, year by year.

On certain evenings — the ones that arrived with a particularly sharp wind, when the sky over the plains grew thin and colorless — he would pause before leaving the lab, turning off the last light with the deliberate motion of someone aware that the work did not end simply because the day did. He would stand for a moment in the doorway, listening to the particular stillness that fills a university after midnight. In that stillness, he imagined the next generation: researchers who would read his studies not with skepticism but with fluency, clinicians who would understand the ratio without having to unlearn a warning, mothers who would feed their children fish without fear.

It was this vision — quiet, unpublicized, entirely unheroic — that sustained him more than any accolade could have. He was not trying to change the world dramatically. He was trying to correct it gently. To return it to itself. To restore the balance that had been there from the beginning, long before warnings were written or policies drafted.

A scientist's legacy is rarely a headline. More often, it is a shift so subtle that only the future can perceive it. He accepted this without complaint. He did not need his name attached to the correction. He needed the correction to reach the unborn.

And so he kept going.

The world was slow to change, but not immovable. It had taken decades to build the superstition; it would take time to unwind it. And he — steady, patient, methodical — had already given the work half of his life. He did not intend to stop now, not when the first glimmers of recognition were beginning to break through the institutional frost.

Because he understood something most people never learn:

If a truth is correct enough, it will eventually outlive the fear that tried to bury it.

There were years when the progress was so incremental it seemed almost static — not because the science was uncertain, but because the world required time to unlearn what it had once accepted as gospel. He grew accustomed to this pace. He understood that institutions move according to their own internal physics, and that even when the evidence is irrefutable, the system will not allow itself to turn until all its unspoken permissions align. This was not resistance; it was inertia, and inertia has its own laws.

In the meantime, he kept refining the work.

Every dataset led to a newer, quieter certainty. Every study reinforced the same proportional truth. Every species examined — from the most humble forage fish to the apex predators of the sea — reproduced the same molecular signature: selenium outpaced mercury in almost every ocean species consumed by humans. The shield held. The architecture stood. The sea, despite the accusations leveled at it, remained a sanctuary rather than a threat.

What frustrated him most was not disagreement — he was accustomed to scientific debate — but the persistence of outdated warnings long after their premises had been undermined. Advisory boards, bound by precedent, continued to issue recommendations based on decades-old interpretations that no longer reflected the current understanding. It was as if time had preserved the caution while preventing the correction.

He often wondered whether the science had simply matured too slowly for the public to keep pace. Or perhaps the public had grown too comfortable with its fears to consider that the danger had been misidentified. Fear has a simplicity that truth rarely matches. To understand the selenium-mercury relationship required nuance. Nuance, in turn, required context. And context required listening — something far rarer than reading.

There were recurring moments that revealed the scale of this challenge. A physician, convinced he was protecting his patients, repeated an outdated warning. A nutritionist declined to recommend fish to pregnant women out of an abundance of caution. A researcher dismissed the selenium hypothesis without having read the full body of evidence. None of these individuals were acting in bad faith. They were acting in continuity with what they had been taught.

He realized then that he was not fighting misinformation; he was fighting inheritance.

Inheritance is harder to correct because it carries the weight of trust. People trust warnings that have been repeated for years. They trust agencies that claim to protect them. They trust the guidance of their doctors. And when that trust is anchored in an error, the correction feels like betrayal rather than enlightenment.

This was the paradox he lived with every day:

To tell the truth was, at times, to ask people to question those they trusted most.

He never expressed frustration openly. Instead, he adapted. He learned to frame the ratio not as a challenge to past warnings, but as a refinement — the natural evolution of science, the update that every discipline undergoes when data reaches a tipping point. His purpose was not to confront. It was to guide. A correction delivered gently travels further than a correction delivered sharply.

He also learned to recognize the subtle signs of progress. A researcher asking a question that would not have been asked ten years earlier. A policymaker reconsidering the weight of a single sentence in a public advisory. A clinician who, for the first time, recommended certain fish to pregnant women rather than warning them away. These moments, small in isolation, formed a constellation when viewed across years.

He understood then that he was witnessing the early phase of a paradigm shift — not announced, not celebrated, but unmistakably underway.

He also knew that large corrections in public health do not begin with announcements. They begin with doubt. Not doubt in the data, but doubt in the inherited narrative. Doubt that opens a tiny seam through which truth can eventually enter.

He did not need victory. He needed that seam.

On certain afternoons, when the winter light felt especially thin and the hallways especially still, he would pause beside the windows overlooking the campus and imagine the future landscape of guidance. He could picture a world in which fish were not feared but understood; in which pregnant women were encouraged — confidently — to seek the nutrients their babies needed; in which the ratio he had studied for decades was not an obscure scientific detail, but a guiding principle in public health.

It would come. Not quickly. Not loudly. But inevitably.

Truth has a way of maturing into acceptance long after its messenger has stopped insisting.

For now, he continued the work. He returned to the lab. He answered the emails. He prepared the next presentation for the next room full of decision-makers. He refined the language to make the complicated simple. He adjusted the charts to ensure clarity. He rehearsed the explanations he knew he would have to repeat again and again.

Because repetition was not a burden to him. Repetition was the method by which truth accumulated its strength.

And slowly — molecule by molecule, study by study, year by year — the world was beginning to lean toward proportion.

There were days when the work felt less like research and more like tending a slow-burning lantern — one that cast only a narrow circle of light in an otherwise darkened field. He carried that lantern from meeting to meeting, year after year, knowing that the illumination it offered was not yet strong enough to change the world, but too important to let go dark. This was not a dramatic burden; it was a quiet one, the kind that settles into a person's life the way winter settles over the plains: firmly, without negotiation, and with a strange kind of dignity.

He once tried to estimate how many times he had explained the same molecular relationship — how many audiences had heard the words selenium and mercury spoken together yet remained unable to grasp the simplicity of their interplay. But counting became pointless. The number did not matter. What mattered was the persistence. Not his own, but the persistence of truth. A truth that refused to be undone by misunderstanding, no matter how often it was overshadowed.

When he presented his findings, he always noticed the same pattern in the room. At first, the audience listened with a kind of guarded curiosity. They had heard fragments of this theory before, enough to find it intriguing but not enough to trust it. Then, as he described the historical studies, the enzyme pathways, the binding affinities, the protective mechanisms, the shift toward recognition would begin. It was subtle — a slight softening in posture, a quiet recalibration of interest. And finally, when he showed the comparative ratios across species, the room would enter a momentary stillness, the kind that occurs when a group realizes they have encountered something that will not fit easily into their existing framework.

But the stillness never lasted. When the presentation ended, the old doctrine — the one that had been built over decades of caution — rose back up like a tide reclaiming the shore.

He understood.

Fear is familiar.

Proportion is foreign.

Fear can be memorized.

Proportion must be understood.

Institutions gravitate toward what they can memorize.

And so he did not resent them. He simply continued the work.

What gave him strength was the knowledge that he was not merely analyzing molecules — he was witnessing a pattern older than human civilization. Long before agencies issued advisories, long before physicians wrote guidelines, long before any of the mechanisms of modern fear had been invented, the sea had already solved the problem. Fish contained the very nutrient required to neutralize the element we feared. The protection had always been there. The misunderstanding had arrived later.

On rare occasions, when the data aligned in a particularly elegant way, he allowed himself a private moment of satisfaction. Not pride — he was never given to that — but gratitude. Gratitude that the biology he studied was coherent. Gratitude that nature had provided a solution long before humans complicated it. Gratitude that the developing brain, so vulnerable, had been given a form of molecular guardianship.

But he also knew that guardianship required recognition.

The fetus cannot ask for selenium.

It cannot defend itself from warnings that remove fish from the diet.

It cannot correct the errors made in its name.

And so the responsibility fell to him — not as a crusader, but as a custodian.

The role shaped his days. It shaped his nights. It shaped the quiet intervals in between. Even when he was not actively running experiments or preparing materials, the work inhabited the edges of his attention. He would be reading a paper and pause when an author repeated the old misconception. He would skim a policy document and see the absence of correction. He would listen to a public health announcement and hear the echo of warnings written before the data existed.

None of this embittered him. It clarified him.

He came to see the world not as an adversary, but as a set of interlocking systems — each with its own limitations, each capable of learning, each requiring patience. In this worldview, no institution was malicious. They were simply slow. Slow to change, slow to adapt, slow to adjust their models when new evidence emerged. And he realized that his work required not confrontation, but endurance.

Endurance became its own kind of expertise. A skill as necessary as any laboratory technique.

He once described the ratio as "the simplest truth I've ever studied, and the hardest truth I've ever watched the world accept." He said it without resentment, only observation. He understood that the world was not rejecting the truth; it was resisting the inconvenience of reevaluation.

And so he remained steady.

Steady in the lab.

Steady in the meetings.

Steady through the years when recognition felt distant.

Steady through the years when recognition began, slowly, to appear.

Because he knew something most people never learn:

The world eventually corrects itself,

but only if someone holds the correction long enough for it to become undeniable.

There were moments — fleeting, rare, but unmistakable — when he sensed the first tremors of institutional reconsideration. They never arrived with fanfare. Institutions do not announce their doubts. They reveal them indirectly, in gestures so small they can be missed unless one has spent years listening for them.

A policymaker asking a second question instead of changing the subject.

A researcher requesting the full dataset rather than the summary slide.

A clinician pausing before repeating the old advisory.

A health organization modifying a single sentence in a document — not enough to alter the guidance, but enough to signal that someone had begun to think.

These were not victories. They were symptoms. Signs that the edifice of inherited caution had begun, at long last, to develop hairline fractures. He watched these moments not with triumph but with recognition, the way a farmer watches the first subtle shift in the soil at the end of winter. It did not mean the thaw had arrived. It meant only that the thaw was possible.

Still, he knew that possibility required stewardship.

He had become a kind of custodian of nuance in a world that preferred absolutes. He saw, with increasing clarity, that his work demanded not only scientific rigor but rhetorical discipline. He had to learn how to speak to audiences who heard the word "mercury" long before they heard anything else. He had to navigate the psychological terrain of fear — a terrain far more treacherous than any laboratory.

He learned to explain proportion before danger.

Selenium before mercury.

Function before fear.

Context before caution.

He knew that reversing an old narrative required creating an intellectual foothold before attempting to shift the entire structure. People needed something to hold onto — not a contradiction, but an evolution. He was not saying the old warnings were irresponsible. He was saying the old warnings were incomplete. Incomplete was a gentler truth, one that allowed people to adjust without feeling deceived.

In time, he realized that correcting a superstition was not an act of confrontation but an act of translation. He was translating molecular reality into institutional language, translating biochemical protection into policy nuance, translating an ancient evolutionary safeguard into something the modern world could trust again.

But translation, even done perfectly, does not guarantee acceptance.

There were years when every meeting felt like a rehearsal of the same polite resistance. And there were years when he suspected the world would always remain two steps behind the evidence. But he also knew something deeper — something that had sustained him through the long winters and the long silences:

Biology does not wait for permission to be true.

Whether the agencies accepted it or not, the ratio remained. Whether the guidelines shifted or not, the protective architecture persisted. Whether the public understood or not, the fetus received its defense from the ocean's quiet generosity.

He found comfort in this constancy.

There were evenings when he left the campus feeling the weight of another unpersuasive meeting, another stalled discussion, another advisory board unwilling to rewrite its narrative. But by the time he reached his car, the wind would have risen — the unmistakable northern wind that carried the scent of the river, the scent of cold, the scent of vast open distances. It reminded him that the work was not about recognition. It was about fidelity. Fidelity to a truth that required endurance more than applause.

The next morning he would return. Not because he was hopeful, but because he was responsible.

Responsibility, he had learned, is quieter than hope but far more durable. Hope can dissolve under discouragement. Responsibility does not. Responsibility endures in the absence of encouragement, in the absence of recognition, in the absence of certainty.

He lived by that endurance.

And slowly — so slowly it would have been invisible to anyone who had not spent decades watching — the world began to shift. A sentence softened. A warning reconsidered. A guideline amended. A new generation of nutritionists emerging without the old fears. A young researcher presenting work that built directly on the ratio, without needing to dismantle old assumptions first.

These were subtle signs, almost imperceptible unless one knew how to look for them. But he knew. He recognized them for what they were:

The beginning of the correction.

Not the correction itself — that would take longer, perhaps decades more — but the first movements of an old narrative acknowledging its own limits.

And in those moments, as brief as they were, he felt something he hadn't expected:

Not relief.

Not victory.

But continuity.

A sense that the work would outlive him, as all true corrections must.

A sense that the world, slow as it was, could still return to its proportions.

A sense that the unborn, one day, would benefit from a truth carried long before they arrived.

It was enough.

And so he continued.

There were seasons — whole stretches of months — when nothing outward seemed to change at all. The advisories remained the same. The pamphlets were untouched. The committees met, adjourned, reconvened, and adjourned again without altering a single clause. To an outside observer, it would have appeared as though the world had rejected his work entirely. But he knew better. He understood that institutions often change long before they admit it. The shift begins quietly, in the unspoken recognition that the old narrative no longer fits as cleanly as it once did.

He could sense this unspoken recognition in unexpected places.

A colleague who had once dismissed his findings began quoting them without attribution — not in malice, but in the natural way people absorb truths they are not yet ready to acknowledge publicly. A graduate student, unaware of the controversy, approached him with a question so informed it could only have come from reading the data firsthand rather than through the filter of inherited warnings. A young researcher from another university expressed interest in studying the ratio, describing it not as an outlier theory but as a "promising direction" in nutritional biochemistry.

These were small things, but they revealed something monumental:

the next generation was not burdened by the assumptions that had constrained the last.

He learned to draw energy from these quiet shifts. Not excitement — he was not given to excitement — but a kind of renewed steadiness. It reminded him that time itself was an ally. The same span of years that allowed a misconception to ossify could, with enough persistence, allow it to soften and eventually dissolve.

He also discovered something else, something he would not have predicted early in his career: the further he advanced into this work, the more the moral dimension revealed itself. This was unusual for a scientist — unusual for him especially — and yet it became impossible to ignore. Science was not conducted in isolation. It influenced the choices of the unborn, who had no voice in the warnings issued on their behalf. And when a warning steered mothers away from the very foods that safeguarded their children's neurological development, the consequences were not theoretical.

There were nights when he sat in his office, long after the last student had left the building, and contemplated this paradox: that the world believed it was protecting the fetus by withholding fish, while in reality it was withholding the protection the fetus needed. The tragedy was not loud. It was quiet, diffuse, almost invisible — the kind of harm that could not be counted, only inferred.

He never allowed these thoughts to harden into anger. Anger would have clouded the clarity of his work. Instead, he allowed them to become fuel — a reminder that the correction mattered not because it was scientifically elegant, but because it was humanly necessary.

One afternoon, late in a winter that seemed determined not to end, he found himself speaking at a small regional conference. The room was modest — a hotel meeting space with dim lighting and a draft most likely caused by a poorly sealed window. There were perhaps twenty attendees, most of them clinicians from rural hospitals. It was not the kind of setting in which one expects to witness a shift in public health understanding.

And yet, something happened there that had eluded him in larger, more prestigious venues.

As he walked them through the selenium-mercury ratio, the expressions in the room did not reflect skepticism or polite discomfort. They reflected recognition. Genuine recognition — the kind that occurs when information aligns with common sense and clinical observation. These clinicians had seen the nutritional deficits that resulted from overly cautious guidance. They had watched pregnant women avoid foods that could have supported fetal development. They had wondered, quietly, if something in the old warnings no longer matched the reality they were seeing.

When he finished, one of the clinicians — an older woman with the kind of clear-eyed steadiness that comes from decades of service — raised her hand and asked, "Why aren't we teaching this already?"

It was not a challenge.

It was not a complaint.

It was a moment of clarity.

And he realized then that the shift would not begin in the large agencies or the national committees. It would begin in rooms like this — small, unadorned, practical. The rooms where responsibility is still felt personally rather than bureaucratically. The rooms where people choose food not from guidelines, but from instinct.

He left that conference with a quiet certainty: the correction was no longer theoretical. It had begun.

Not everywhere.

Not fully.

But undeniably.

The superstition was cracking.

The ratio was entering the world.

And the unborn — slowly, gradually, inevitably — would one day receive the protection they had been denied.

He walked back to his car through the brittle cold, the sun already low on the horizon, and for the first time in many years, he felt not continuity but acceleration — the faint but unmistakable sense that the world had finally begun to move.

There is a moment in every long struggle when the resistance that once felt immovable begins to lose its density. It does not collapse. It does not admit defeat. It simply thins, almost imperceptibly, like ice growing translucent before the first thaw. He felt this thinning not in the grand arenas of policy — those would be the last to shift — but in smaller, human moments that revealed a quiet reordering of thought.

A letter from a clinician he had never met, thanking him for clarifying something she had always suspected intuitively.

A brief mention in a research paper that treated the selenium-mercury ratio not as a fringe finding but as an emerging principle.

A call from a nutritionist seeking advice not because she doubted him, but because she wanted to present the information accurately to her patients.

These were not transformations. They were confirmations — signs that the truth had begun to embed itself in the places where sincerity outweighed procedural caution.

He understood then that change does not begin where authority resides.

It begins where responsibility resides.

And responsibility, he knew, lived closer to the ground — in the hands of physicians who delivered children, in the kitchens of families, in classrooms where future clinicians learned how to think about risk and nutrition. These were the places where the old warnings caused the most unintended harm. These were the places where a correction would matter most.

He had always believed that the truth of the ratio was too elegant to remain in obscurity forever. What he had not anticipated was how unevenly the correction would travel. Some communities, especially those familiar with the nutritional realities of pregnancy, embraced the new understanding readily. Others clung to the old warnings with near-religious devotion, as if to revise them were to invite a kind of ancestral disloyalty.

It was in these environments — the ones where fear had calcified — that he exercised his deepest patience. He never confronted. He never contradicted directly.

Instead, he offered the molecular architecture with the same steady calm he had maintained for decades. He knew that anger would be interpreted as arrogance, and arrogance would poison the message. By contrast, clarity — the quiet, disciplined kind — had a way of softening resistance.

But even with this patience, there were moments when the weight of the work pressed against him. Not because he was discouraged, but because he could see, with painful clarity, the cost of delay. Every year the old advisories remained in place was another year of children developing without the full benefit of omega-3s — another year of mothers choosing safety at the expense of necessity. The harm was never dramatic. It was cumulative, dispersed, almost invisible. He carried the knowledge of that harm with the same gravity that defined his research.

Occasionally, he would sit alone in his office late at night, long after the campus had emptied, and reflect on the strange shape his career had taken. When he began, he had not imagined that his life's work would be devoted to correcting a misunderstanding. Most scientists chase novelty, innovation, discovery. He found himself chasing accuracy — not a new truth, but a long-neglected one. There was a humility in that pursuit, but also a kind of quiet nobility. He was not advancing a theory. He was repairing a narrative.

What surprised him most was how much of this work took place beyond the reach of scientific journals. The journals were necessary — foundational, in fact — but they were not sufficient. The true battleground was in the public mind, the policy documents, the medical advice given in exam rooms. It was in the places where fear had been legitimized. And so he learned to speak not only as a scientist, but as a communicator.

He never adopted theatrics. Never adopted the sensational language that often propels ideas into public consciousness. He spoke instead with the same clarity that governed his research — calm, measured, proportionate. The irony was not lost on him: he was trying to correct a fear-based narrative using the language least likely to bypass fear.

But he trusted the intelligence of those who listened.

He trusted time.

He trusted the molecules.

On a particularly cold evening, when the wind over the river carried the metallic scent of deep winter, he paused before entering the lab and watched the lights inside flicker against the glass. There was no drama in the scene, no symbolism he could articulate, yet something in that moment crystallized: an understanding that the work had never truly been about recognition or institutional acceptance. It had always been about fidelity to a truth that predated him and would outlast him.

He stepped inside and closed the door behind him.

The world was moving — slowly, hesitantly, imperfectly — but moving nonetheless.

And the correction, once unthinkable, had already begun its long emergence.

There is a point in any long endeavor when the work begins to shape the worker, not through revelation but through the slow accumulation of discipline. He had entered the field as a scientist, trained to look outward — toward data, mechanisms, enzymatic behaviors — but over the years, the work had begun to turn inward.

Not in a self-absorbed way, but in the sense that he had become attuned to the internal mechanics of patience, clarity, restraint. His temperament, already steady by nature, had settled into a kind of quiet inevitability.

He no longer questioned whether the world would accept the truth. He questioned only when.

It was this temporal distinction — not if, but when — that carried him through the years when nothing visible seemed to change. Progress was not linear. It was recursive. A movement forward, then a period of stillness. A glimmer of recognition, then silence. A promising discussion, then months of bureaucratic immobility. But beneath this surface drift, he could sense a deeper shift — not in policy, not in guidelines, but in the intellectual climate itself.

People were beginning to entertain the possibility that the fear had been misplaced.

He saw it in the way questions were asked, the way assumptions were tested, the way younger researchers approached the material without the preloaded caution that had defined the earlier generation. They were curious rather than defensive. Open rather than anchored. They did not carry the psychological residue of the old warnings. To them, the ratio was not subversive. It was sensible.

This generational difference did not make him optimistic in the naïve sense. He did not believe change would arrive suddenly or completely. But he recognized that the intellectual soil had begun to loosen. The old roots, once immovable, were losing their grip.

This realization brought him a sense of quiet steadiness — not excitement, but assurance.

He had learned, over time, to measure progress not by declarations but by patterns. And the patterns were unmistakable. Papers that once ignored the ratio now included it. Agencies that once dismissed the significance of selenium now referenced it, albeit cautiously. Health organizations softened their language, shifting from absolute warnings to risk-based nuance. It was not the revolution some might expect. It was something more enduring: the slow reorientation of a field toward proportion.

He also began to understand something deeper, something almost philosophical: the work was not only about fish, or nutrients, or fetal neurodevelopment. It was about the psychology of fear and the cost of overcorrection. It was about how societies protect themselves — sometimes wisely, sometimes recklessly. It was about the fragility of truth when it is competing against a narrative designed to soothe rather than illuminate.

He knew that the original mercury warnings were issued with sincere intentions. They were attempts to protect the fetus from a toxin that, in certain contexts, could indeed cause harm. But caution, once institutionalized, tends to drift into absolutism. The nuance dissolves. The proportions disappear. And what remains is a monolithic warning — broad, blunt, uncalibrated.

He was trying to restore calibration.

Not to overthrow the warning, but to refine it. To make it accurate. To ensure that protection did not become deprivation. To ensure that the unborn were not shielded from a toxin at the cost of the nutrient that shielded them from it.

On certain evenings, when he paused between tasks and let his eyes rest on the horizon through the lab window, he felt a sense of something he could not quite name — not pride, not weariness, but an awareness that he was part of something larger than himself. A continuity that stretched backward into the history of scientific correction and forward into a future where the error he had spent his life addressing would be remembered not as a scandal, but as a transitional misunderstanding.

This was the nature of his legacy — quiet, methodical, unceremonious.

He did not imagine his name would be celebrated, nor that the correction would be attributed fully to him. Science does not honor its patient custodians loudly. But he took comfort in knowing that, long after he was gone, children would develop with stronger neurological foundations because their mothers had been given better guidance. The recognition would not be his. The benefit would be theirs.

And that, he understood, was the only form of permanence that mattered.

He returned to his desk, adjusted a stack of papers, and began preparing for the next day's work — another set of samples to analyze, another set of questions to answer, another room to sit in with individuals who were still learning to understand what he had seen so clearly for so long.

He did not resent the slowness of progress.

He expected it.

He respected it.

He endured it.

And as he worked, the thought settled again — soft, steady, certain:

The correction was no longer a possibility.

It was a trajectory.

There were periods when the work seemed to exist in two parallel worlds — the world of molecular truth, which was precise and unwavering, and the world of public interpretation, which shifted according to preference, pressure, and precedent. He learned to navigate both without allowing the dissonance to erode his clarity. The truth was steady. The world was not. His task was to serve the truth long enough for the world to catch up.

This dual existence shaped him in unexpected ways. It made him more observant, more attuned to the subtleties of human hesitation. He began to notice how often people deferred not to knowledge, but to comfort. How frequently decisions were made not from evidence, but from the psychological need to maintain a consistent narrative. How a warning, once repeated, became a kind of cultural artifact — resistant to revision, even in the face of data.

He also noticed something else: most people did not reject his findings because they doubted the science. They rejected them because the correction required them to admit that a fear they had carried — and taught — might have been misplaced. People resist being wrong far more than they resist being uninformed. It was this distinction that clarified his strategy. He would not ask the world to renounce its earlier caution. He would ask it only to refine it.

Refinement, he knew, was far easier to accept than reversal.

One morning, during a lecture at the university, he found himself watching the faces of the students as he explained the molecular mechanism. They listened not with suspicion, but with curiosity — the unburdened curiosity that comes only from those encountering a subject without inherited anxiety. These students had grown up in a world where nutritional advice was ubiquitous, often contradictory, and therefore less sacred than it had been to earlier generations. They were open to complexity. They were open to correction. They were open in ways that their mentors had struggled to be.

It occurred to him then that the future of his work did not lie solely in policy change, but in intellectual succession. A new generation of scientists, clinicians, and policymakers would eventually take their place in the institutions that had resisted him. And when they did, they would carry none of the defensive habits that had kept the ratio from entering the mainstream. They would treat it as intuitive — perhaps even obvious.

This realization did not lessen the urgency of his work, but it gave him a second horizon. The first horizon was institutional acceptance — slow, resistant, procedural. The second was generational — fluid, fertile, inevitable.

He worked toward both, knowing that the latter would succeed even if the former lagged.

With this perspective, he began to move through his days with a calmness that was almost architectural. He no longer viewed each meeting as a referendum on his life's work. He viewed each as a brick laid in a structure that would eventually support the correction. Even when he encountered the same objections, the same reluctance, the same polite deferrals, he saw them as features of a system protecting its past, not rejecting its future.

This clarity brought a kind of inward spaciousness. He could hold the slowness without resentment, hold the resistance without frustration, hold the setbacks without self-doubt. The work was larger than any single moment, and certainly larger than any single meeting. He had grown into the patience his work required.

One evening, as he walked across the campus parking lot, the sky had deepened into that vast, slate-blue quietness characteristic of the northern plains. There was no sound except the soft crunch of snow under his boots. He paused halfway to his car, noticing how the lights from the science building cast long, clean lines across the ground. He stood there for a moment, absorbing the stillness, and felt something rare: an awareness that he was exactly where he needed to be.

The world would change — slowly, unevenly, imperfectly — but it would change.

And when it finally did, the correction would seem so logical that people would wonder why it had taken so long. They would assume it had always been known. The ratio would be taught as if it had never been contested. The warnings would be revised quietly, without ceremony, as though the revision had been inevitable all along.

He would not be credited for this inevitability. That was not how scientific corrections were remembered. But the unborn — those voiceless recipients of his entire career — would inherit the benefits of the truth he had held through decades of winter.

This was the work.

This was the meaning.

This was enough.

There were stretches of time — sometimes a month, sometimes a season — when his days settled into a rhythm so subtle it barely registered as routine. He would arrive at the lab before the first hint of sun cleared the horizon, unlocking the building with the quiet familiarity of someone who had spent more hours inside its walls than outside them. He had walked those halls in every state of weather: blizzard mornings when the sky felt close enough to touch, thawing afternoons when the river began its slow release, dry summer nights when the prairie held the faint scent of dust and grass. Through all of it, the work remained constant — patient, unhurried, unyielding.

He never framed these years as sacrifice. Sacrifice implies something offered in exchange for reward. He asked nothing in return for his endurance. The reward, if it existed at all, lived far beyond him — in the minds of future mothers who would one day make decisions with better knowledge, in the bodies of children whose earliest neural architecture would be supported by nutrients long misunderstood. The work was its own justification.

He knew — perhaps more clearly than anyone else — that most scientific careers are not defined by grand discoveries but by the slow accumulation of clarity. And clarity is rarely dramatic. It emerges gradually, in the same way dawn emerges on the northern plains: not as a sudden illumination, but as a quiet surrender of darkness. His findings had followed that same arc. Each study, each dataset, each recalculated ratio brought him closer to a truth he had felt long before he had fully articulated it.

But even clarity had its burdens.

The more deeply he understood the biochemical reality, the more acutely he felt the distance between truth and practice. It was not enough to know the fetus required the nutrients in fish. He had to watch, year after year, as public guidance unintentionally discouraged the very foods that protected the developing brain. It was not enough to understand the selenium-mercury relationship. He had to witness, in silence, the consequences of a warning repeated without revision.

There were moments when that distance — between what was true and what was believed — felt almost like a physical weight. He never allowed the weight to show in his demeanor. He remained steady, reserved, unassumingly observant. But if one looked closely, there were signs: the brief pause before answering a question he had answered a hundred times before; the slight tightening around his eyes when someone cited the old warnings; the way his gaze sometimes drifted to the window, as if the horizon might offer an explanation the institutions could not.

Still, he never lost faith in the eventual correction.

He believed, quietly but firmly, that the truth possessed a structural integrity that could not be undone by misunderstanding. Error required reinforcement; truth required only time. The world could misinterpret mercury, misapply caution, misalign its warnings — but none of that altered the molecular reality he had spent his life studying. Selenium continued to protect the brain. Fish continued to carry that protection. The fetus continued to depend on it.

No advisory, however well-intentioned, could rewrite the biology.

That constancy gave him strength.

He knew that the correction would not come as a sweeping reform. It would arrive piece by piece, in the way most corrections do: a revised paragraph in a medical curriculum, a footnote in a policy document, a clinician adjusting their dietary recommendations, a young researcher repeating the ratio in a seminar without realizing its history. Corrections rarely announce themselves. They appear, quietly, in the margins of practice.

What mattered was that he remained present long enough to shepherd the transition.

He once confided — in a rare moment of candor — that he wished he could speak directly to the unborn children his work was meant to protect. Not to explain the science, but to assure them that someone had been watching closely, paying attention, ensuring that the mistakes of the past would not be repeated indefinitely. It was not a sentimental impulse. It was an expression of responsibility — the purest form of it.

He was not their advocate in any official sense. He held no public office, oversaw no agency, revised no national guidelines. And yet, in a deeper sense, he was their guardian — not of their lives, but of the information that would shape those lives before they were even capable of knowing it.

This understanding — quiet, unspoken, unpublicized — became the compass of his work.

And so he continued, not for recognition, not for approval, not for vindication, but because he understood the stakes with a precision the world had yet to internalize. He carried the ratio the way one carries a vital instrument — carefully, attentively, aware that someday, someone else would inherit its meaning.

The winters passed. The advisories lingered. The studies accumulated. The world moved slowly.

But truth — patient, molecular, incorruptible — remained exactly where he had found it.

There were winters when the cold seemed almost sentient — a presence that settled into the bones of the university itself, pressing against the windows with the steady insistence of something testing the integrity of a structure. He never minded those winters. In a strange way, he preferred them. The cold simplified the world. It stripped everything down to what could endure. In that stripped-down landscape, his work felt less like an anomaly and more like a natural fit: something patient, persistent, resilient enough to withstand seasons of silence.

He often thought that if the general public could see science the way the northern plains experienced winter, they might understand why the correction took so long. Winter does not end because the calendar demands it. It ends because the accumulated weight of cold eventually gives way to the accumulated pressure of light. In the same way, misconceptions do not dissolve because one scientist presents clearer data. They dissolve only when the accumulated weight of error can no longer withstand the pressure of truth.

He had become intimately familiar with that pressure.

It was there in every conversation where he sensed a flicker of recognition behind someone's cautious expression.

It was there in every dataset that reinforced the molecular architecture.

It was there in every question from a student who approached the material without inherited fear.

It was there in every small alteration to institutional language — not enough to be noticed publicly, but enough for him to recognize as evidence of a slow internal shifting.

And it was there, most powerfully, in the knowledge that even if the institutions lagged, the molecules did not.

That constancy — the unwavering logic of selenium protecting the brain from mercury — became the fixed point around which he arranged his entire understanding of the world's resistance. When confronted with skepticism, he reminded himself: the fetus still receives protection from selenium. When discouraged by an unchanged advisory, he reminded himself: the ratio still holds in every species studied. When frustrated by the inertia of institutions, he reminded himself: the developing brain still depends on what the sea provides.

The truth had survived decades of misunderstanding. It could survive a few more.

He knew, of course, that most people never glimpsed the magnitude of the correction he was trying to shepherd. They saw only a dietary recommendation, a line in a pamphlet, a cautious sentence offered in a doctor's office. They did not see the quiet tragedy behind those sentences — the subtle deprivation occurring at the molecular level when a mother avoided fish during pregnancy. They did not see how a single misunderstanding repeated for decades could echo through a generation's neurological development.

He saw it.

Not abstractly, but concretely — in data points, in biochemical pathways, in epidemiological patterns.

He had studied the consequences long enough to recognize their shape.

But he never judged the public for its fear. Fear is the simplest form of protection. It costs nothing intellectually. It is easy to memorize and easy to repeat. The truth he carried, however, required discernment. It required a willingness to think in ratios rather than absolutes, in relationships rather than binaries. It required the kind of mental discipline that most people were never trained to exercise. And so he offered the truth patiently, knowing that the world's resistance was not defiance but unfamiliarity.

He could remember, with surprising clarity, a meeting early in his career when a senior official, after listening to him explain the ratio, asked, "Why haven't we heard this before?" He responded with the calmness that had already begun to define him: "Because we weren't looking in the right direction." It was the closest he ever came to criticism. Even then, his tone carried no accusation — only proportion.

As years passed, that proportion became his signature — not in the public sense, but in the moral sense. He approached every conversation, every presentation, every written explanation with the same disciplined steadiness. He believed that tone was as important as data. Tone determined whether the truth could enter a resistant mind. Tone determined whether the correction felt like an attack or an evolution. Tone determined whether people could walk away feeling enlightened rather than embarrassed.

He had learned the hard way that people protect their reputations with more ferocity than they protect the truth. And so he approached reputations with respect — even those that had inadvertently prolonged the misunderstanding.

But he never softened the truth itself.

The fetus needed fish.

Fish carried selenium.

Selenium neutralized mercury.

The architecture was complete.

The danger lay not in consumption, but in avoidance.

He carried these sentences not as slogans but as a kind of molecular ethics — a responsibility he had inherited by virtue of understanding something the world had not yet fully absorbed.

And he kept going, through winters and thaws, through years of resistance and years of subtle progress, always returning to the same quiet conviction:

A truth this clear did not require victory.

It required endurance.

There were days when he moved through the university with the instinctive quiet of someone who had learned to inhabit the margins of an institution without ever demanding its attention. Not because he felt out of place, but because he understood that the work he carried did not require an audience — only continuity. He walked the same hallways season after season, his presence becoming as steady and unobtrusive as the radiators humming against the winter cold. People greeted him with the polite warmth reserved for familiar figures whose significance is felt more than spoken.

He never needed the institution to acknowledge him to know he belonged to it. Belonging, he had learned, was not bestowed by recognition but earned by persistence. And persistence was the one currency he possessed in abundance.

He often reflected on how strange it was that the world could misinterpret the very foods that had sustained it for centuries. Human history had been inseparable from the sea. Entire civilizations had risen along coasts, nourished by the reliability of fish, strengthened by its nutrients during the most fragile stages of development. Then, in a single generation, fear had disrupted that lineage. A warning — issued before the full proportion was understood — had overshadowed millennia of biological wisdom.

He wondered whether the sea itself would have found the irony amusing. The ocean had done nothing differently. Its fish still carried the selenium that protected human neurodevelopment. Its food chain still enforced the same biochemical patterns. The misunderstanding had not come from the sea. It had come from humanity's tendency to interpret danger in isolation rather than in relationship.

He had spent years trying to articulate this distinction: mercury was not the danger; imbalance was.

He repeated this idea so often that it became a kind of internal monologue, present even when he was engaged in unrelated tasks. It accompanied him as he sorted through sample data, as he reviewed manuscripts, as he answered emails from researchers wanting clarification. It accompanied him in the quiet intervals of his life — on walks across campus, on late-night drives home, on the rare evenings when he allowed himself the small luxury of reading something unrelated to his work.

And in these intervals, when the world felt momentarily still, he would allow himself to think about the deeper implications of the misunderstanding. How many decisions were made each day based on inherited caution rather than informed discernment? How many mothers altered their diets out of fear rather than proportion? How many clinicians repeated warnings not because they believed them, but because they could not risk deviating from institutional scripts?

He had once believed that expertise alone could correct a misconception. With time, he realized that misconceptions were not rooted in ignorance but in narrative. The mercury warning had become a narrative — one that offered a sense of control, a sense of protection, a sense of moral responsibility. To challenge it was not merely to present new data; it was to ask people to reexamine their own identity as caregivers, protectors, advisors.

This insight taught him restraint.

He never framed the correction as a repudiation of earlier guidance. He framed it as an evolution — a natural refinement that accompanied scientific progress. He spoke gently, because the truth, delivered gently, traveled further. And yet, beneath that gentleness, he carried a steel-edged clarity. He could not compromise the science. He could not dilute the truth to spare institutional feelings. He could only present it in a way that preserved dignity for those who were hearing it for the first time.

This balance — uncompromising accuracy delivered with unassuming grace — became the defining characteristic of his work.

He suspected few people recognized how deliberate it was. They saw the calm, the patience, the quiet manner of speaking, and assumed it was merely personality. They did not see the intentional discipline behind it — the way he had shaped his tone to carry a truth that required years of repetition to penetrate layers of inherited caution.

He had learned something most scientists never confront: that the truth is not rejected because it is incorrect, but because it is inconvenient.

And yet, he remained unmoved by this inconvenience. Not stoic — stoicism is a posture. His steadiness was not postured. It was organic, the natural result of someone who believed deeply in the moral necessity of his work. He did not need recognition. He needed the world to stop depriving the unborn of the nutrients that safeguarded their development. That was all.

There were evenings — especially in the depth of winter — when he would walk past the empty lecture halls and feel the faint echo of his own lectures lingering in the air. Not the words themselves, but the questions they had raised. He imagined the students carrying those questions into their futures, into their careers, into the clinics and labs and policy rooms where they would one day work. He imagined them speaking of the ratio not as an anomaly, but as a foundation. And he felt, in those moments, a quiet assurance that the seeds he had planted were already germinating.

He never expected to witness the full transformation. That was not how scientific corrections worked. They unfolded across decades, carried by people who inherited the truth without inheriting the struggle it took to reveal it. He was comfortable with that anonymity. He was comfortable knowing that the future would move forward without ever needing to know how many winters he had spent holding the line.

Because the line had held.

And that was enough.

There were mornings when he arrived on campus before the first custodial lights flickered on, when the world still felt unclaimed and the sky had not yet decided whether it would offer sun or surrender to another gray expanse. These early hours were not an escape — they were a sanctuary. The silence of the building, the faint hum of ventilation systems, the echo of his footsteps in the long hallways — all of it formed a kind of private prelude to the day's work. In that quiet, the complexity of the world fell away, leaving only the precision of the molecules he studied.

In those moments, he often reflected on how strange it was that the simplest truths required the most endurance. The selenium-mercury ratio was not mysterious. It did not demand speculative leaps or revolutionary instruments. It revealed itself through patient observation and disciplined inquiry — the kind of science that grows incrementally, like rings in a tree. Yet this simplicity had made it harder, not easier, for the world to accept. People expect threats to be straightforward, not balanced by counterforces. They expect danger to act alone, not in dialogue with its counterpart. They expect toxins to be vanquished, not neutralized.

But biology is a conversation, not a monologue.

He had spent much of his life trying to teach the world this distinction: that mercury's danger was contextual, not absolute. That selenium was not merely beneficial, but protective. That fish were not vectors of harm, but carriers of equilibrium. And that the fetus — so fragile, so dependent — required not protection from the sea, but partnership with it.

Yet for years, his words had entered a world that preferred singular warnings to relational truths. Warnings were easier to print, easier to teach, easier to enforce. A sentence that said "avoid fish" fit neatly into a pamphlet. A sentence that said "consume fish with adequate selenium to support neurodevelopment and counter mercury's binding preferences" did not.

He knew this.

He understood the psychology.

He understood the bureaucracy.

He understood the cultural momentum of fear.

And still, he persisted.

Not because he believed he could overturn the world's caution with a single lecture — he knew better than that — but because he understood that corrections accumulate the same way misunderstandings do: slowly, almost invisibly, one repetition at a time.

He had seen this pattern before. In graduate school, in earlier research fields, in the incremental shifts of scientific understanding. Breakthroughs are remembered as singular events, but they are almost always the result of years of quiet recalibration. He had come to see the entire field of nutritional toxicology as a system that needed recalibration — not overthrowing, not refuting, not humiliating — just recalibrating.

He sometimes imagined what the world would look like if the correction were complete — if the warnings aligned with the molecular reality, if clinicians confidently explained the relationship between selenium and mercury, if expectant mothers chose fish not with fear but with purpose. In that imagined world, his decades of work would appear small, almost trivial — a simple refinement. That is the paradox of success in fields like his: the more fully a correction is adopted, the less visible the struggle behind it becomes.

He was at peace with that paradox.

Visibility had never been his currency.

Accuracy was.

Integrity was.

Patience was.

He had cultivated these qualities the way others cultivate ambition — not as a performance, but as a necessity. He knew that endurance was the only tool capable of outlasting institutional inertia. He knew that calm was the only tone capable of entering rooms where fear dictated the conversation. He knew that clarity was the only bridge between biochemical truth and public understanding.

This clarity shaped him in ways he rarely acknowledged, even to himself. It gave him a sense of proportion not only in science, but in life. He moved through the world with an understanding that everything was relational — not only mercury and selenium, but truth and time, effort and outcome, work and recognition. He viewed progress not as something that could be demanded, but as something that emerged when the conditions were right — when the intellectual climate had thawed enough to allow new understanding to take root.

He had not reached that point yet, not fully. But he could sense the thaw beginning — in the cautious questions, in the revised drafts of policies, in the murmuring interest of younger researchers. The world was not rejecting the truth. It was preparing for it.

And he, ever patient, ever steady, remained exactly where he needed to be:

at the threshold of the correction, holding the door open until the world was ready to walk through.

There were stretches of late afternoon when the light in his office took on a kind of muted gold — the hour when the sun angled low across the plains and the shadows of the window frames lengthened across his desk. In that hour, the campus often felt suspended between two worlds: the outward-facing bustle of academia and the inward-facing silence of research. He preferred the latter. It was in these quiet intervals, when the building exhaled the last remnants of daytime noise, that he often understood the work most clearly.

Not the data — he always understood the data — but the meaning.

Meaning did not arrive in the laboratory. It arrived in the stillness afterward, when he could look at the day without urgency and recognize the shape of what he was doing. In those moments, he sometimes felt as though he were translating two separate languages that had not yet learned to speak to each other: the language of molecules, precise and unyielding, and the language of institutions, cautious and reluctant.

He had become fluent in both.

This fluency did not come quickly. At the beginning of his career, he spoke only in the language of science — ratios, pathways, affinities, oxidative stress, enzymatic function. It was enough to communicate with peers, but not enough to shift the broader world. Over time, he learned that the public does not accept truth because it is true; it accepts truth because it becomes comprehensible. And comprehension requires narrative — not storytelling, but structure.

So he began to shape the science into a structure the world could hold.

He spoke of balance.

He spoke of proportion.

He spoke of the developing brain as a sovereign architecture requiring specific materials.

He spoke of selenium not as a trace nutrient but as a guardian.

He spoke of mercury not as a singular toxin but as a rival.

He spoke of fish not as hazards but as vessels of equilibrium.

He never dramatized.

He never exaggerated.

He never adorned the truth.

He simply shaped it.

And slowly, the world began to listen — not because the science had changed, but because the way he carried it had.

People trusted him not because he preached, but because he explained. They trusted him not because he led with certainty, but because he led with proportion. He spoke calmly in a landscape saturated with anxiety, and in that calmness, people found something they could lean into.

He understood, perhaps earlier than most, that fear does not dissolve under pressure. It dissolves under understanding. Pressure only cements it further. Understanding requires time — and time requires patience.

Patience had become the quiet backbone of his life.

It was evident in everything: the way he paused before answering a question; the way he arranged his papers meticulously, not out of compulsion but clarity; the way he gave his full attention to people who had dismissed him previously, as though he believed—sincerely—that every conversation was a new opportunity to begin again.

In that patience, something remarkable occurred: he stopped anticipating resistance. He simply expected the world to take the time it needed. And once he removed anticipation from his posture, conversations began to unfold differently. People felt less threatened. Less defensive. More curious. His calmness became a kind of permission — permission for others to reconsider what they had assumed was settled.

He realized, eventually, that this was how truth entered systems resistant to revision: not with force, but with readiness.

And readiness, he knew, was arriving.

It arrived in the language of young scientists who no longer felt the need to defend the old warnings. It arrived in the questions of clinicians who wanted to protect their patients more accurately. It arrived in the tentative shifts within agencies that had once been immovable. It arrived in the slight, almost imperceptible changes in tone — from certainty to inquiry, from caution to calibration.

These were the sounds of a field thawing.

One evening, as he walked across the nearly empty parking lot, he noticed a thin line of melting snow running along the edge of the pavement. The temperature was still cold enough to keep the ground frozen, yet the sun had lingered just long enough that day to alter the surface. A small shift, almost invisible. But unmistakable.

That was the nature of his work.

That was the nature of correction.

That was the nature of truth when it begins to prevail.

He watched the thin line disappear beneath the fading light, and he understood — with a clarity that felt both earned and effortless — that he no longer needed to wonder whether the world would change.

It had already begun.

There were evenings when the campus felt almost impossibly still — not empty, but suspended, as if the world were holding its breath in the narrow space between what had been believed and what would eventually be understood. He grew familiar with that stillness. In time, he even came to depend on it. The work required a particular kind of quiet: not silence, but mental unencumbrance — the freedom to think in ratios when the rest of the world still thought in warnings.

It was in that quiet that he often recognized how deeply the misunderstanding had woven itself into culture. Fear had not merely shaped advisories; it had shaped identities. Expectant mothers took pride in avoidance, believing restraint equaled protection. Clinicians took pride in guidance, believing caution equaled vigilance. Policymakers took pride in issuing warnings, believing oversight equaled safety. The mercury narrative had not been a simple misinterpretation — it had been a moral posture.

He understood then that his true adversary was not misinformation.

It was certainty.

Certainty — that most seductive of human comforts — was far harder to correct than ignorance. Ignorance invites learning; certainty resists it. And certainty wrapped in the language of responsibility becomes nearly unassailable. He had entered a field where caution had been elevated to virtue, and where virtue had become immune to revision.

This realization might have discouraged another man.

It steadied him.

Because he understood something most people never pause long enough to see: certainty is fragile. All it takes is one undeniable truth — repeated patiently, carried steadily, delivered without accusation — to begin the unraveling. Not a confrontation. Not a refutation. A quiet, persistent presence.

He became that presence.

He noticed, over time, how often people would lower their defenses when he spoke. Not because he softened the truth, but because he refused to frame it as a challenge to their integrity. He never asked anyone to admit they had been wrong. He asked only that they look again. He had a way of offering truth that preserved dignity on both sides — a skill far rarer, and far more essential, than most people realize.

It was this quality — more than the data, more than the publications, more than the presentations — that allowed the correction to begin.

He had learned that scientific revolutions do not occur when the evidence becomes irrefutable. They occur when the evidence becomes undeniable and the messenger becomes unthreatening.

It was no small thing to carry a truth that required decades of repetition. It demanded stamina — intellectual, emotional, moral. It required an ability to be both persistent and patient, both precise and gracious. It required the discipline to present the same findings year after year, knowing that understanding would bloom not through argument but through accumulation.

In these years, he discovered something unexpected: the longer he carried the truth, the less it felt like a burden and the more it felt like a form of stewardship. A truth this elegant — this protective, this ancient, this quietly benevolent — deserved a custodian who would not distort it for persuasion, dramatize it for attention, or weaponize it for ego.

He became such a custodian almost unintentionally, through temperament rather than ambition.

And the longer he held the truth, the more he realized that the world would not resist forever. It couldn't. Fear may travel quickly, but proportion travels faithfully. And faithfulness, in the end, always outlasts alarm.

One late night, walking between buildings as snow drifted in slow spirals under the yellow lamplight, he paused at the sight of a single set of footprints — his own — trailing behind him in an unbroken line. Without meaning to, he wondered if this was what his career looked like: a solitary track stretching across a vast, indifferent landscape.

But the thought passed as quickly as it arrived.

Because he knew better.

The track was not solitary. He had walked it long enough that others were beginning to follow. Slowly. Tentatively. Curiously. But following nonetheless.

He turned toward the darkened building where his office light still glowed — a small square of yellow in the winter dusk — and he felt, not pride, but continuity: the sense that the work was no longer just his to carry. The path he had carved was becoming visible.

The correction had roots now.

There were seasons when he sensed the shift not in headlines or policy drafts, but in subtler, more intimate signs — the kind of signs that only someone who had lived with a truth for decades could recognize. A question asked differently. A hesitation where certainty had once been. A clinician phrasing a recommendation in a way that suggested they were no longer convinced by the original warning. These were faint signals, easy to overlook, but he registered each one with the quiet acuity of someone who had trained himself to hear what others dismissed as background noise.

He had grown accustomed to listening for change in places where change rarely announced itself.

He knew that institutions often spoke in coded language long before they altered their official positions. A shift in tone preceded a shift in policy. A shift in emphasis preceded a shift in guidance. A shift in what people no longer said often mattered more than what they did. And so he paid attention not only to the presence of misconceptions, but to their gradual erosion — the way certain phrases began to disappear from discussions, the way certain assumptions no longer appeared unquestioned.

To him, these omissions were as telling as data points.

He remembered a particular advisory meeting — one of countless he had attended — where the customary phrase "avoid fish during pregnancy" did not appear even once. The committee had not replaced the warning with a revised statement, nor had they acknowledged the omission. They simply did not repeat the old guidance. It was as if the narrative had loosened its grip just enough to create an opening, a brief moment of intellectual oxygen. He left the meeting not triumphant, but aware: something had shifted.

That was how paradigms began to turn — not with declarations, but with absences.

He learned to inhabit these absences with care. He never pressed harder when he sensed a rhetorical softening. He allowed the new space to widen naturally. He understood that too much pressure could cause institutions to retreat, to re-entrench themselves in the familiar. But a gentle presence — a steady repetition of proportion, a calm articulation of molecular reality — could expand the space gradually, almost imperceptibly.

This was the art within the science: the ability to apply exactly the amount of pressure the moment could bear.

Over time, he realized that the resistance he encountered was not a wall but a membrane — pliable, responsive, capable of yielding when approached with the right balance of clarity and patience. When he spoke with frustration, the membrane thickened. When he spoke with precision, it thinned. He refined his tone accordingly, not as performance but as recognition of the work's psychological dimension.

He had become, in effect, a diplomat on behalf of the molecules.

This role surprised him. He had never thought of himself as a negotiator. But he found that the ratio required him to negotiate not between opposing parties, but between truth and fear — a negotiation as old as humanity itself. He did not choose sides. He did not condemn caution. He simply insisted on proportion, the one principle that undergirded every biological and ethical dimension of his work.

One late winter afternoon, after a particularly long meeting, he walked out onto the frozen path behind the science building and paused at the edge of the river. The ice was beginning to fracture — not dramatically, but subtly, in thin lines that caught the low light. He crouched to examine a fissure, tracing the pattern with his eyes. It was not a break; it was the beginning of movement.

He felt in that moment a recognition so instinctive it did not require words:

the world was beginning to crack in the right places.

Not collapse — crack.

Not shatter — shift.

Not overturn — unfreeze.

It was all he had ever wanted.

Not vindication. Not victory. Not acclaim.

Just movement — honest, proportionate movement — in a direction aligned with the truth.

He stood slowly, brushed the snow from his gloves, and felt a quiet conviction: the correction was no longer confined to the lab or to the meetings or to the minds of a few open-hearted clinicians. It was beginning to seep outward, to migrate into the culture of guidance. The membrane was thinning. The river was loosening. The narrative, once frozen, was beginning to flow.

And he understood, as he turned back toward the building, that the next phase of the work would not require more force, but more constancy — the same steady presence that had carried the first twenty years would carry the next.

He walked back inside, the door closing softly behind him.

There were moments — sparse, almost fragile — when he allowed himself to imagine what the world might feel like once the correction was complete. Not in grand terms, not in sweeping reforms or celebratory declarations, but in the quiet ways everyday life would change. A clinician speaking with unburdened confidence instead of caution. An expectant mother choosing fish without fear. A medical student learning the ratio as foundational knowledge rather than revisionist detail. These were the kinds of futures he pictured, and they were modest enough to be believable.

But he never lingered there long. Imagination was not where his work lived. His work lived in the unglamorous present — in the slow accumulation of clarity, the daily discipline of patience, the fidelity to a truth that could not be hurried.

Still, he recognized that imagining the future gave shape to the present. It reminded him why he remained steady even when the world resisted clarity. It reminded him why the long hours in the lab mattered, why the endless meetings mattered, why the gentle tone mattered. It reminded him that the correction was not theoretical — it was eventual.

There was a particular day — he never marked the date, but he remembered the light — when he felt the future draw closer. He had been invited to speak at a gathering of young nutrition researchers, most of whom had grown up with the old warnings but were no longer beholden to them. They were curious in the purest sense: unthreatened by contradiction, unburdened by institutional loyalty, unconcerned with defending inherited errors.

He began the lecture as he always did, with proportion rather than alarm. He explained the ancient biochemical relationship, the elegance of selenium's affinity, the way the ocean had arranged itself to protect the developing brain long before humans developed language to describe it. As he spoke, he sensed something unusual. The room was not resisting. It was leaning forward.

When he finished, a young woman near the front raised her hand and asked, "Why hasn't this been the standard explanation all along?"

He paused for a moment, recognizing the same question he had heard years earlier from a clinician in a rural conference room — but this time, the tone was different. It wasn't frustration. It wasn't confusion. It was simply incredulity: the incredulity that arises when the obvious has been obscured for too long.

This, he realized, was the moment when the generational threshold had been crossed.

The correction was no longer his alone. It had begun to embed itself into the intellectual reflexes of people who would one day lead the field. It no longer rested solely on his decades of endurance. It had entered the bloodstream of a new scientific culture.

He left that lecture with a sense of something rare — not relief, not triumph, but recognition. Recognition that the truth had finally acquired momentum. Recognition that the next generation would carry it without the burdens he had borne. Recognition that the world had begun to tilt, almost imperceptibly, toward proportion.

And yet, even as the momentum increased, he did not allow himself to withdraw from the work. Momentum does not replace stewardship. If anything, it makes stewardship more necessary. He remained careful, deliberate, intentional in every explanation he offered. He continued refining his language, not to persuade those who resisted, but to guide those who were newly receptive. He understood that the transition from misconception to understanding required a steady hand — someone who could translate the science without diluting it, who could steward the ratio through its final stages of acceptance.

He returned to his office that evening and sat for a long time without turning on the light. The room was washed in the pale glow of the winter dusk, the kind of light that softened the edges of everything — the papers on his desk, the framed certificates on the wall, the quiet instruments resting in their places. The building hummed around him, familiar in a way few places in life ever become.

He felt, in that moment, a calm that was deeper than satisfaction. It was the calm of someone who understood that the hardest part of the journey was behind him. The world was no longer solid ice. It was thawing. Not evenly, not everywhere, but undeniably.

And he knew, with a clarity he had not possessed in his earlier years, that the remaining distance — however long — would unfold on its own terms.

He would walk it.

Not to force the correction, but to accompany it.

There were days when the pace of the world felt misaligned with the pace of his work — the world always straining toward immediacy, toward announcements and breakthroughs and visible transformation, while his work moved according to the slow, internal rhythm of biological truth. He never envied the velocity of other fields. Velocity was fragile.

It burned brightly and disappeared quickly. What he carried required durability, not spectacle.

He understood that he was engaged in a form of science that demanded the same patience as geology — shifts measured not in moments, but in seasons, layers, and sediment. Human understanding, he often thought, resembled sediment more than structure: it accumulated gradually, compacted over time, resistant to disturbance, yet vulnerable to subtle pressures.

He had become one of those pressures — not disruptive, not forceful, but steady.

He learned long ago that his influence did not lie in persuasion. Persuasion implied a contest, and contests implied victories and losses. His work was not a contest. It was a calibration. A return to proportion after decades of imbalance. A rediscovery of what had always been true. Biology did not change. Only interpretation did.

What surprised him most, as the years passed, was how much of the misunderstanding had been rooted not in malice or incompetence, but in fear. Fear had shaped entire advisory structures. Fear had constructed narratives that felt protective, even when they caused harm. Fear had overridden proportion, because proportion requires trust — trust in complexity, trust in nuance, trust in the idea that danger is rarely absolute.

He never condemned the fear. He simply refused to inherit it.

His days unfolded with a kind of disciplined serenity. Even when meetings grew tense, even when colleagues questioned the ratio with tone rather than evidence, even when policy boards deferred decisions again and again, he maintained a demeanor that felt almost architectural — constructed deliberately, with clean lines and quiet weight.

He understood that people listened not only to what he said, but to how he bore the truth he carried.

When he spoke without urgency, they felt less urgency.

When he spoke without defensiveness, they felt less threatened.

When he spoke without frustration, they felt less obligated to resist.

Calm became its own form of instruction.

He did not design it that way. It happened naturally, a consequence of living with the truth long enough that it shaped his temperament. The ratio had taught him something profound: that balance is not the absence of conflict but the steady presence of counterforces. Selenium and mercury did not cancel each other; they competed. They interacted. They revealed something essential about the world: danger is contextual. Protection is relational. And understanding requires seeing both at once.

He brought this philosophy into every conversation. When someone expressed concern about mercury, he did not dismiss the concern; he contextualized it. When someone insisted that the original warnings were necessary, he did not contradict them; he expanded the frame. When someone clung to certainty, he offered proportion. And in doing so, he became, quietly, a model of the very principle he was trying to teach.

One late afternoon, as he was packing up his notes from a day of meetings, a colleague lingered in the doorway. She was someone who had once been skeptical — not hostile, just anchored in the old narrative. She hesitated for a moment before saying, "I've been thinking about what you said last month. I think..." She paused, searching for the right phrasing. "...I think I may have oversimplified the risk."

He nodded gently, offering no triumph. "It's an easy risk to oversimplify," he replied.

Her shoulders eased. She smiled — a small, almost embarrassed smile — and said, "Thank you for being patient."

He knew what she meant. She wasn't thanking him for the science. She was thanking him for the manner in which he carried it — the quietness, the steadiness, the refusal to turn the correction into a confrontation. That moment, more than any citation or acknowledgment, affirmed the moral architecture of his work.

After she left, he sat alone for a moment, absorbing the weight of that exchange. Not because it marked a victory, but because it marked a shift — a human shift, the kind that could not be mandated by policy or induced by data alone. It was the kind of shift that signaled readiness.

He gathered his things, turned off the desk lamp, and stepped into the hallway. The building was quiet, the long corridor illuminated by the muted fluorescence of nighttime energy-saving lights. He walked slowly, unhurried, attuned to the subtle echo of his footsteps. The stillness felt familiar, almost companionable.

As he pushed open the door to the outside, a rush of cold air met him — sharp, immediate, unmistakably northern. He breathed it in deeply, letting the clarity of the cold settle into his lungs. The sky above him was a deep, clean blue, the kind that appears only in late winter when the horizon sharpens against the coming thaw.

The world was changing.

Slowly.

Quietly.

Proportionately.

And he knew — with the same certainty he felt when interpreting a dataset, with the same calm that had carried him through decades of resistance — that he would continue walking this path until the correction no longer needed him.

He stepped into the cold evening, the door closing softly behind him.

There were phases of the work — long ones — when he no longer measured progress by what anyone said aloud. Words, he had learned, were unreliable indicators of change. They arrived too early, or too late, or carried more caution than conviction. Instead, he measured progress by the quiet reorientations in people's behavior, the subtle reorganizing of what they paid attention to, what they questioned, what they no longer defended.

It was in these behavioral shifts that he detected the earliest signs of a new intellectual climate.

For years, whenever he presented the molecular architecture of selenium and mercury, audiences would instinctively brace themselves at the mention of "mercury." Shoulders tightened. Pens paused. Expressions sharpened into a familiar posture of alarm. But recently, he noticed that this reflex had softened.

The word no longer carried the same immediate theatricality. A few listeners still reacted out of habit, but many simply leaned in as if waiting for nuance rather than danger.

This, to him, was extraordinary.

Fear, once embedded in a culture, is almost impossible to unseat. It becomes a moral reflex — a signal of vigilance, a badge of conscientiousness. Yet here it was, loosening. Not dramatically, not across the entire field, but in pockets. Pockets that would eventually widen into corridors, and corridors that would eventually widen into a new standard.

He understood better than anyone that scientific corrections begin as murmurs before they ever become doctrines.

There was a complexity in the air now — a willingness to consider proportion, to ask questions that would have been unthinkable a decade earlier. He saw it in how researchers framed their hypotheses, in the kinds of variables clinicians now requested in studies, in the way policy analysts examined historical advisories with a more critical lens.

Even the tone of institutional correspondence had changed. Once-uncompromising statements now included clauses like "emerging evidence suggests..." or "the balance of nutrients may warrant further review..." These were not admissions, but they were openings. And openings, he knew, were more valuable than declarations.

He never mistook these shifts for resolution. He understood that the old narrative still held enormous psychological weight. But he also understood that such weight was beginning to redistribute — subtly, like the first internal movements of a glacier long before anyone sees the ice break.

He felt these internal movements in unexpected moments.

A colleague who had dismissed him years earlier now sent a paper with the note, "Thought this might interest you."

A policymaker asked him to review a draft not because she agreed, but because she wanted to "avoid oversimplification."

A young researcher, unburdened by the old caution, used the phrase "selenium adequacy" as if it were ordinary parlance — as if it had always belonged in discussions of neurodevelopment.

These moments were imperceptible to the world, but unmistakable to him. They indicated that the correction had entered a middle stage — the stage where a truth stops being resisted and begins being quietly absorbed.

He once described this stage, privately, as "the silent uptake." It was the phase when people internalized the logic before they adopted the language. They acted with proportion before they spoke with proportion. Understanding precedes articulation. This, he believed, was how real change occurred — not by proclamation, but by osmosis.

He carried this awareness with the calmness of someone who had watched entire seasons pass without a single visible sign of progress. Now, the signs — however faint — were present, and he recognized them with the precision of a scientist and the intuition of someone who had held the truth long enough to feel its movements instinctively.

On a quiet evening, he stepped out of the building just as the sun was setting. The air had begun to soften — not warm, not yet, but less severe. The sky held a pale gradient of color, not quite gold, not quite gray. He paused for a moment, letting the cool air settle around him, and he sensed something he rarely allowed himself to acknowledge:

the beginning of relief.

Not relief from the work — the work was ongoing, and he would continue it as long as he could — but relief from the isolation that had defined his earliest decades. The truth no longer lived solely in his hands. It had spread, not explosively, but faithfully, like warmth returning to frozen ground.

He walked toward his car as the horizon dimmed, aware that the world was not fully changed — but it was no longer unchanged.

And in that distinction — subtle, precise, unmistakable — he felt the quiet promise of what was still to come.

There were days when the work felt almost weightless — not because its burden had diminished, but because he had grown so attuned to its cadence that carrying it no longer required conscious effort. He had become, in a sense, indistinguishable from the work itself. The ratio lived in him the way language lives in someone who has spoken it since childhood: fluently, instinctively, without hesitation. He no longer rehearsed explanations. He simply articulated what he knew, and the clarity followed.

Yet even in this fluency, he remained careful.

Clarity, he understood, could be mistaken for certainty if delivered without humility, and certainty — the wrong kind — had been the root of the original misunderstanding. So he continued speaking with the measured tone that had become his signature, conveying not urgency, but inevitability.

He knew that inevitability was often the most persuasive form of truth.

One morning, during a routine departmental seminar, he listened as a younger colleague presented research that indirectly supported the ratio. The colleague did not mention him by name, nor did he reference the history of the field. He simply explained the biochemical mechanism as though it were established — as though it had always been taught this way. The room absorbed the information calmly, almost casually. There were no raised eyebrows, no objections, no defensive questions.

It was the ordinariness of the moment that astonished him.

Ordinariness is the final stage of acceptance.

When a truth stops sounding new, it stops sounding controversial.

When it stops sounding controversial, it becomes infrastructure.

And when it becomes infrastructure, it becomes permanent.

As he watched the presentation unfold, he felt a quiet sense of displacement — not the painful kind, but the kind that accompanies a transition into legacy. The truth no longer needed him as its sole advocate. It had found new custodians: people who did not carry the scars of earlier resistance, who did not associate the ratio with controversy, who approached the science without the emotional architecture that had shaped its earliest debates.

He sat back slightly in his chair, folding his hands, and allowed himself a small, inward breath. Not satisfaction — something deeper. Continuity. The knowledge that the baton had begun to pass, not because he had relinquished it, but because the field had finally grown into it.

On his walk back to the lab, he thought about how differently this moment would have felt if it had occurred twenty years earlier. Back then, he might have viewed it as validation or vindication. Now, it felt more like witnessing the natural evolution of something he had tended for so long that it had become its own organism.

He had allowed the truth to mature without forcing it, and now it was maturing without him.

As he reached his office, he noticed a stack of student papers on his desk — assignments from a course he had taught quietly for years. He sorted through them with the calm precision of someone who understood the significance of shaping young minds not through persuasion, but through exposure. One paper in particular caught his attention. A student had written:

"The protective role of selenium suggests that earlier guidelines may have overlooked the relational nature of nutrient interactions. Future advisories should reflect this proportion."

He read the sentence twice. It was not dramatic. It was not embellished. It was not a manifesto. It was a simple, elegant statement — the kind of statement that only appears when understanding has moved from concept to intuition.

He placed the paper gently on top of the pile.

He often wondered whether the world would ever fully recognize the decades he had spent holding the line against silence, inertia, and fear. But moments like this — quiet, unpublicized, almost private — assured him that recognition was irrelevant. Understanding was what mattered. And understanding was taking root precisely where it needed to: in the minds of people who would carry it forward without hesitation, without trauma, without the long shadows of earlier debates.

The next phase of the correction would not require confrontation.

It would require integration.

He leaned back in his chair for a moment, letting the steady hum of the building settle around him, and felt the quiet satisfaction of someone who has lived long enough within a truth to see it begin to live without him.

The work was no longer fragile.

The field was no longer frozen.

The narrative was no longer singular.

And he understood — with a calm that felt earned, seasoned, inevitable — that what remained was simply to continue, with the same steady presence that had carried the first twenty years into the next.

There were mornings when he sensed, even before entering the building, that the work had entered a new phase — a phase defined not by resistance or persuasion, but by a wider, quieter form of recognition. It did not arrive as praise, nor as institutional endorsement. It arrived as alignment. The world was beginning to tilt toward the truth, not dramatically, not all at once, but unmistakably.

This shift revealed itself in subtle ways. A visiting researcher would reference the ratio in passing, as though it had always been part of the standard framework. A clinician from another state would request clarification not because they were skeptical, but because they wanted to integrate the science responsibly into patient guidance. A public health advisor would cite emerging patterns in nutritional outcomes that aligned perfectly with what he had been saying for years.

The tone of these interactions had changed.

Less guarded.

Less defensive.

Less burdened by the legacy of the original warning.

It was as though the field itself had exhaled.

He noticed that people no longer approached him with the brittle caution reserved for those who challenge doctrine. Instead, they approached him with the easy respect reserved for someone whose work had become foundational. They no longer treated the ratio as an anomaly. They treated it as a lens — a way of seeing the world that clarified much of what had previously seemed contradictory.

This was the quiet triumph of proportion: it made things make sense.

He had spent decades living inside that clarity, and now, slowly, others were entering it as well. In their questions, he heard the early echoes of the future — the kind of future where nutritional guidance would be shaped not by fear, but by fidelity to biochemical reality. It was a future where clinicians would speak of fish with calm confidence, where expectant mothers would receive recommendations rooted in proportion rather than anxiety, where policy documents would reflect the actual relationship between nutrients rather than the imagined conflict between them.

The work was becoming architecture.

One afternoon, as he prepared for a seminar, he found himself reflecting on the arc of his career — not with nostalgia, but with the sober clarity of someone who had been present for every stage of the correction. He thought of the early years, when even speaking about the protective role of selenium felt like stepping into a headwind. He thought of the middle years, when small victories often arrived disguised as ordinary conversations. And he thought of the present, when the boundaries of the field had quietly expanded to accommodate the truth he had carried alone for so long.

He realized something then — something he had felt but never articulated:

the correction was no longer a possibility.

It was a culture.

The realization settled over him with a calm, steady warmth.

He walked into the seminar room, where a group of graduate students were already gathered. They were talking quietly, comparing notes, adjusting their laptops. He listened for a moment before beginning, and in their voices — unburdened, curious, confident — he heard the unmistakable sound of a generation that would inherit the truth without the resistance that had shaped his own path.

When he began to speak, he noticed something he had never noticed so clearly before:

they understood him not as a messenger of controversy, but as a messenger of clarity.

The ratio was not an argument.

It was an understanding.

And understanding, once established, needs no defense.

As he walked back to his office afterward, he passed a display case in the hallway containing photographs of researchers from earlier decades — people whose work had once seemed controversial, disruptive, even unwelcome, but who were now remembered for their fidelity to truth, not for the resistance they endured. He stopped in front of the case for a moment, studying their faces, and felt an unexpected sense of kinship.

He wondered if anyone would ever place his photograph there.

It didn't matter.

Ultimately, the molecules kept their own memory.

He continued down the quiet hallway, his footsteps echoing softly, and reached his office just as the sun was beginning to set. The light fell across his desk in long, warm bands, illuminating the papers, the graphs, the quiet instruments that had shaped decades of understanding. He sat for a moment, hands resting on the edge of the desk, and felt something he had not allowed himself to feel for many years:

the early form of closure — not an ending, but the beginning of one.

Not because the work was finished, but because the world had finally begun to carry it with him.

The hallway outside was silent.

The building felt steady.

The truth felt permanent.

There were evenings when the building itself seemed to hold its breath, as though it understood that some transitions must occur in quiet rather than proclamation. He felt the shift most acutely in these intervals — the hours after the daily movement of the campus had dissolved into a hush, when the fluorescent hallway lights hummed with their familiar low timbre and the outside world receded into a blue-grey calm.

He often paused at his office door during these hours, not out of hesitation, but out of recognition. The threshold marked more than the boundary between corridor and workspace; it marked the boundary between two eras of his own understanding. There had been a time when he entered this room with the weight of being an outlier. Now he entered with the awareness that the field had begun to reshape itself around the truth he had carried.

It was not victory.

It was not triumph.

It was alignment — the most dignified of all outcomes.

He settled into his chair, listening to the faint heating system murmuring through the vents, and allowed himself a rare acknowledgment: the misalignment that had once defined the narrative was slowly dissolving. Not through confrontation, but through quiet absorption. The field was recalibrating itself exactly as biology recalibrates — gradually, proportionately, through internal correction rather than external force.

He had always believed that clarity, once revealed, possessed its own momentum. Proportion was not an argument; it was a gravity. And gravity, once established, does not ask permission. It simply asserts itself through inevitability.

One day, while reviewing a new manuscript submitted for peer commentary, he noticed something striking — not in the data itself, but in the framing. The authors referenced selenium's protective role as a given, not a hypothesis. They treated it not as a challenge to existing guidance, but as an integral component of nutritional understanding. The ratio had moved from the margins into the architecture of explanation.

He sat back, holding the manuscript lightly in his hands, and experienced an inward stillness so complete it felt like the room itself had shifted. He realized that this was the moment every long-arc scientist hopes for but rarely witnesses: the moment when the truth becomes unremarkable.

Unremarkable, he knew, was the highest form of acceptance.

Remarkable truths require defense.

Unremarkable truths require only recognition.

He closed the manuscript gently, as though it were a fragile artifact of a future he had been preparing for decades, and he felt the unmistakable sensation of arrival — not his arrival, but the arrival of the correction itself.

It took root without ceremony.

It embedded itself without announcement.

It lived now in places he would never see.

Later that week, he found himself walking through the cafeteria — a place he visited rarely — and overheard two students discussing dietary guidance for pregnancy. One of them mentioned selenium as though it were common knowledge, weaving it seamlessly into a broader conversation about nutrient interactions. There was no hesitation, no defensiveness, no sense that the idea carried history or controversy. It was simply part of their intellectual landscape.

He did not stop. He did not introduce himself. He did not intervene or correct or guide. He simply walked past, his footsteps quiet on the linoleum floor, carrying an awareness that the work had begun to live independently of him.

That, he understood, was the purest form of legacy.

Not statues or awards or recognition.

Not citations or headlines or acknowledgments.

Legacy was continuity — the moment when the truth no longer needed him as its voice.

He returned to his office with this realization settling over him in slow, steady layers. He sat down, adjusted the papers on his desk, and experienced the rare, grounding sensation of a responsibility finally beginning to redistribute itself. The weight he had carried for so long had not disappeared — it had simply become shared.

He looked out the window at the soft blue dusk gathering across the campus, and he felt the quiet satisfaction of someone who had spent decades walking into headwinds only to discover, at last, that the wind had shifted direction.

Not completely.

Not uniformly.

But undeniably.

And in that shift, he sensed the early formation of something deeper than closure — something like inheritance. The truth, once fragile, was now being carried by others with a steadiness that matched his own.

The night settled over the plains, subtle and unhurried.

He gathered a few papers, untouched by urgency, and turned off the lamp.

There were long stretches of late winter when the horizon over the plains held a kind of austere clarity — the kind that reveals not beauty but coherence. He found himself drawn to that coherence more and more in these later years of the work. It mirrored something he had begun to feel within himself: a settling, a gradual alignment between what he knew, what he had endured, and what the world was finally beginning to understand.

It was an unexpected feeling — not triumph, not relief — but something quieter, deeper, and more rare:

vindication without spectacle.

He had never imagined the correction would arrive with fanfare. The misalignment had been too old, too comfortable, too deeply woven into institutional posture for that. But he also knew the correction would not be silent. When truth enters a system that has lived with error for a generation, it alters not the surface, but the internal geometry.

He was beginning to see those geometric shifts everywhere.

A dean who once avoided eye contact when the ratio was mentioned now greeted him with the easy respect reserved for someone whose contributions had been quietly reassessed.

A policy researcher who had dismissed him years ago now asked for a meeting, not to debate but to understand.

A scientific board that once sidestepped the topic now requested updated language "to ensure accuracy."

The shifts were subtle, but unmistakable.

People were not admitting the old narrative had been wrong — institutions rarely grant such clarity — but they were behaving as though the correction had already taken place.

This behavior fascinated him.

It was confirmation that the field had reached its inflection point: the moment when belief no longer needed announcement because it had already migrated into instinct. He recognized it the way a seasoned navigator recognizes a change in the wind — not by sound or sight, but by the faint pressure of air against the skin.

He found himself reflecting on the strange symmetry between the science he carried and the social landscape through which he carried it. Selenium's role was protective, not aggressive. It did not attack mercury; it constrained it. It did not eradicate danger; it balanced it.

His entire career had become an echo of that principle.

He had not confronted institutions; he had constrained their errors.

He had not dismantled fear; he had balanced it with proportion.

He had not demanded recognition; he had allowed understanding to accumulate in the right places, at the right pace.

In this way, he had become the human analogue of the very element he studied — a quiet guardian, a counterforce, a stabilizing presence in a landscape vulnerable to imbalance.

He felt this most clearly one afternoon when he hosted a small workshop for public health students. They were attentive in the way young people often are — earnest, curious, unburdened by the hierarchies that shape their elders' thinking. They asked precise questions, not performative ones. They listened without suspicion.

One of them, a soft-spoken young man, stayed afterward to thank him.

"I think the way you explained this," he said, "makes more sense than anything I've read in the guidelines."

It was not the words that struck him — students often expressed appreciation — but the tone. It wasn't admiration. It was comprehension. The kind of comprehension that indicated these students would never again view fish through the lens of inherited fear. They had encountered proportion early, before the old narrative could calcify in their thinking.

Later, as he walked across the parking lot, he thought of how many years it had taken to reach a moment like that — a single sentence spoken by someone who would someday influence others, spoken without controversy, spoken without hesitation, spoken as though the truth had always been obvious.

He paused beside his car, watching a thin veil of snow drift across the asphalt, and he felt an odd, quiet gratitude — not for recognition, but for the small fact that the next generation would not have to unlearn what their predecessors had been taught. They would begin from a place of proportion rather than distortion.

This, he realized, was the essence of the work:

not correcting the past, but protecting the future.

Not persuading the reluctant, but preparing the receptive.

Not dismantling fear, but outlasting it.

He unlocked the car, settled into the driver's seat, and rested his hands on the steering wheel for a moment before starting the engine. Outside, the wind stirred lightly, carrying with it the early signs of a season shifting toward spring — the slow thaw, the subtle drift, the soft erosion of winter's authority.

The world was changing.

The truth had taken root.

The correction was no longer an argument, but an inheritance.

He exhaled once, slowly, and let the quiet fill the space around him.

There were nights when he lingered in the parking lot longer than necessary, the engine still quiet, the keys cold in his hand, as though some part of him needed a few extra moments to absorb what the day had revealed. These pauses were never planned. They simply happened — small pockets of stillness between the lab and the road, between the work and the rest of his life. In these moments, he often found himself contemplating not the science, but the strange temporal geometry of influence.

It occurred to him, more than once, that the correction he had carried for decades was no longer moving at his pace. It had begun to move at its own.

This realization surfaced in ways that were almost too quiet to articulate. A former skeptic forwarding him an article "you might find interesting," even though the article supported what he had been saying for twenty years. A policy draft arriving in his inbox with a note that read, "We're considering adjusting the language — would appreciate your perspective." A clinician he barely knew recommending one of his papers to a colleague without realizing he was within earshot.

None of these gestures were grand.

None were dramatic.

But each one represented a subtle, dignified shift in the world around him.

He had learned to read these shifts as clearly as he read analytical charts — not by their volume, but by their consistency. When the same quiet signals began appearing across different contexts, he knew the field had entered its irreversible stage: the point where the truth no longer needed defense because it had begun to shape the intellectual instincts of others.

He felt this most profoundly one afternoon during a meeting with a small advisory committee. It was a modest gathering — a rectangular conference table, a few pitchers of water, a handful of neatly printed agendas. He had attended countless such meetings, many of them strained by the tension between institutional caution and biochemical reality. But this one felt different before it even began. The air in the room held a strange lightness, the kind that precedes the softening of a long-held position.

Halfway through the meeting, someone — a senior official known for her adherence to established guidelines — said something so subtle and unexpected that he almost missed its significance.

"I think we may have overemphasized the risk," she said, glancing at her notes. "The nutrient balance deserves more weight than we've historically given it."

The statement was not framed as a confession. It was framed as a refinement — the kind of refinement that appears only when institutions are preparing themselves for revision. There was no defensiveness in her tone, no deflection. Just a straightforward acknowledgment that proportion had been neglected.

He did not respond immediately. He allowed the sentence to rest in the air, to be absorbed by the others in the room. When he finally spoke, he did so with the quiet steadiness that had become his constant posture.

"It's an easy balance to overlook," he said. "But once you see it, it's impossible to unsee."

The room was silent for a moment. Not tense — reflective. A silence that marked the beginning of consensus rather than the absence of it.

When the meeting adjourned, he walked down the long corridor toward the exit, the soft glow of overhead lights casting elongated reflections on the polished floor. As he passed the glass cases filled with the history of the department, he felt a shift inside himself as well — not pride, but perspective. He realized that he had been present for the entire arc of a misunderstanding: its rise, its entrenchment, its slow unraveling, and now its quiet correction.

He stepped outside into the early evening calm. The air was cool but no longer severe — the sort of air that suggests winter is preparing to leave even if the calendar refuses to confirm it. A thin crescent moon hung low over the prairie, faint but precise, like a small incision in the sky.

He stood there for a moment, watching the horizon settle into its blue-violet hush, and felt the strange, almost tender recognition that the work was no longer solitary. The understanding had migrated outward. It lived now in the minds of others — clinicians, students, researchers, policymakers — people who would carry it into rooms he would never enter.

The truth had grown roots and branches and new custodians.

He inhaled the evening air slowly, letting the quiet expand inside him, and then unlocked his car with a single, unhurried motion.

The world was still imperfect.

The work was still unfinished.

But the trajectory was no longer in doubt.

He started the engine, the headlights cutting a clean path across the dimming lot, and he felt — for the first time in many years — that the long corridor ahead was no longer uphill.

There were mornings when the world felt newly arranged, as if the plains themselves had shifted during the night and the university sat a fraction of an inch closer to some unseen horizon. He could never explain this sensation fully — it wasn't tied to weather, or the season, or even his own mood. It was something subtler, something atmospheric: the feeling that the work had advanced again, not through any visible milestone, but through a quiet reconfiguration of how people thought.

He had come to recognize these mornings as markers.

Not of victory, but of inevitability.

They arrived without warning and without ceremony. He would unlock his office, hang his coat on the same peg, set his notebook on the same desk, and yet feel — unmistakably — that something in the intellectual climate had warmed by a single degree. A sentence spoken differently the day before. A question asked with a new tone. A hesitation replaced by curiosity. The smallest shifts, but all pointing in the same direction.

This was how paradigms changed: not with earthquakes, but with pressure.

He had once believed that understanding required force — a decisive correction, a definitive statement, a single moment of clarity that would cause the old warning to collapse. But the longer he lived with the truth, the more he understood that paradigms dissolve not through confrontation, but through accumulation. A single truth repeated gently for long enough becomes indistinguishable from common sense.

And common sense requires no defender.

It was during one of these quietly altered mornings that he received an email from a research institution overseas — a place that had historically echoed the strictest interpretations of the old mercury guidance. The message was brief, almost perfunctory:

"We are revising our maternal nutrition recommendations and would appreciate your perspective on integrating selenium-related considerations."

He read the sentence twice.

Not because it was surprising — the shift had been gathering for years — but because of its tone. It was not skeptical. It was not hesitant. It was not framed as a debate. It was written with the calm assumption that his perspective was necessary, perhaps even foundational.

For the first time, the question was not whether the world should recalibrate.

The question was how.

He drafted his response with the same steady cadence that had carried him through earlier decades — precise, proportionate, unadorned — and as he typed, he felt a subtle yet unmistakable quiet settle over him. It was the quiet of someone who no longer needed to push. The world was leaning toward him now, not away from him.

That afternoon, he found himself in the lab analyzing a new series of samples. It was work he had done thousands of times — methodical, repetitive, almost meditative. As he moved through the familiar procedures, he realized how profoundly the work had shaped him. Patience had become not just a tool but a temperament. Clarity had become not just a goal but a way of seeing. And proportion — the guiding principle of the ratio — had become the logic through which he understood everything.

Even time.

Time itself had become a kind of element, one he had learned to work with rather than against. Early in his career, he had felt the weight of urgency — the need to correct, to persuade, to accelerate the shift. But now, standing at the lab bench with the soft hum of equipment around him, he recognized that urgency had no place in this kind of work. The truth had its own tempo. The world, once resistant, was beginning to match it.

Later, as he walked across campus, the wind carried the faint scent of oncoming thaw — that early, almost poetic signal that winter's authority was beginning to weaken. The river, still frozen, had darkened along its edges, an early sign of movement beneath the surface. He paused on the pedestrian bridge and leaned slightly against the railing, watching the faint shimmer beneath the ice.

That shimmer felt familiar.

It was the shimmer of the correction — not visible, not dramatic, but present.

Alive.

Moving.

He stood there for a long moment, letting the horizon settle around him, and thought about the long arc of the misunderstanding he had spent his life addressing. He thought about the early frustrations, the middle years of incremental gains, the recent shifts in tone and behavior. And he felt — not sentiment, not nostalgia — but clarity.

The truth had outlasted the fear.

The proportion had outlasted the warning.

The molecules had outlasted the misunderstanding.

He turned toward the campus buildings again, their windows glowing softly in the late afternoon light, and walked back with the steady, unhurried gait of someone who no longer questioned the direction of the world's movement.

It was moving toward him now — not because he pushed, but because the truth pulled.

The corridor ahead was open.

The light was increasing.

The work was entering its final, quiet phase.

There were conferences — many of them — where he stood at a podium facing an audience of clinicians, researchers, policymakers, and nutrition advisors from across the world. The locations changed — London, Tokyo, São Paulo, Vancouver, Sydney — but the pattern never did. No matter how advanced the institution or how accomplished the attendees, there was always a portion of the room that looked at him with the tentative curiosity of people encountering a truth they had not known existed.

It was almost always the same proportion: a quarter of the room.

Twenty-five percent.

Not hostile.

Not skeptical.

Simply unaware.

He came to recognize that expression — the slight narrowing of the eyes, the brief pause in note-taking, the visible shift in posture as someone realized that the narrative they had inherited might be incomplete. Sometimes it was a young researcher hearing the molecular relationship for the first time. Sometimes it was a seasoned clinician who had spent decades repeating cautionary phrases crafted in another era. Sometimes it was someone who had simply trusted the old guidance without ever knowing it had been built on incomplete assumptions.

He never judged the gap.

He simply observed it.

Because that 25% represented something important — not resistance, but latency.

They were not defenders of the old propaganda; they were its unknowing heirs.

He understood the dynamics well. A narrative rooted in fear spreads quickly. A narrative rooted in proportion spreads slowly. Fear requires no understanding. Proportion requires discipline. And propaganda — even well-intentioned propaganda — has a way of persisting long after its usefulness has expired.

He learned, over time, to address that 25% with a particular tone — calm, inviting, almost architectural. He did not rush them through the science. He guided them gently, allowing the structure of the molecules to reveal the truth in its own time. He had discovered that the human mind absorbs new understanding not at the pace of information, but at the pace of trust.

And trust had to be earned from people who had been taught to fear the very foods that protected the unborn.

What fascinated him most was that the remaining 75% — those who had heard of the ratio, those who had perhaps begun to integrate it into their thinking — often watched the newly awakened minority with a kind of quiet recognition. As though they too remembered when the truth first unsettled them, when the narrative first cracked, when the possibility of proportion first revealed itself as something sturdier than the old warnings.

The room, in these moments, became a kind of microcosm of the global shift itself:

a majority beginning to move, a minority still catching up, and all of it unfolding slowly — slower than truth deserved, but faster than error wanted.

He never resented the pace.

He respected it.

Because if proportion were something the world could adopt instantly, it wouldn't be proportion. It would be fashion. And fashions disappear. But corrections that take decades to arrive tend to stay.

He left each international presentation with the same quiet understanding:

that the progress of truth is not measured by how many have heard it, but by how many carry it after hearing it for the first time.

And even in those rooms — even when the 25% looked unsettled or uncertain — he felt the slow, steady unraveling of the old propaganda, thread by thread, question by question, mind by mind.

The correction was still slow.

But it was no longer still.

There were gatherings — grand, international, meticulously organized — where he stood on stage beneath polished lights and behind a lectern bearing the emblem of whatever global institution had summoned the world's nutrition authorities for another yearly reassessment of what the public should or should not eat. These events were always the same in their choreography: a procession of credentials, a recitation of acronyms, a reverent tone that hovered somewhere between scientific solemnity and bureaucratic theatre.

And yet, amid all that ceremony, the moment he began to speak, he could feel the divide in the room as clearly as if it were marked on the floor.

The 75% who had at least heard the truth in some form — fragmentarily, cautiously, distantly — and the 25% who had not.

He could identify the latter group instantly.

They leaned forward, not out of interest, but out of orientation. They were positioning themselves inside the lecture, trying to understand its shape. Their eyes did not yet hold recognition; they held recalibration. They held that subtle tension a person experiences when they realize the conceptual ground beneath them may require rearrangement.

He never viewed these listeners as behind.

He viewed them as uninitiated.

Because what they had inherited was not knowledge, but momentum — the momentum of decades-old warnings that had taken on a moral quality, warnings spoken with the conviction of institutional righteousness and repeated by individuals who believed deviation from the script was a breach of duty. These attendees were not defenders of propaganda. They were simply unaware that the propaganda had a half-life.

He spoke to them with a particular kind of discipline: slow, precise, unhurried. He did not rush the molecules. He let selenium reveal itself the way clarity always reveals itself — gently, steadily, proportionately. He did not position mercury as a villain; he positioned it as a participant. A force in dialogue with another force. A toxin whose power was not absolute but contextual.

He could always tell the moment the 25% began to understand.

It happened when their shoulders eased. When their pens resumed movement. When their expressions shifted from vigilance to inquiry. They were not agreeing; they were absorbing. That was enough. Agreement could come later. Absorption was the first threshold.

What struck him every time, no matter the city or the institution or the language through which the question was asked, was how universal the awakening looked. The recalibration of fear into proportion had the same facial expression everywhere on earth. It was as though the world — every corner of it — was wired to recognize balance once balance was finally shown.

And yet, even as he watched these small awakenings unfold, he never forgot that the 25% represented something deeper than ignorance: they represented the world as it had been for most of his career.

They were the living archive of the imbalance he had spent decades correcting.

After each presentation, during the mingling sessions where professionals gathered in small clusters holding paper cups of coffee, he would inevitably be approached by one or two members of that uninitiated quarter. They always spoke with the same combination of politeness and humility, the kind that arises when someone suspects that their training may have missed something essential.

“I hadn’t heard this before,” they would say.

Or, “Why wasn’t this part of my coursework?”

Or the most honest and most common:

“How long has this been known?”

He always answered gently.

“Long enough,” he would say, “that

There were conferences where he could feel, within minutes of beginning his remarks, that the room was unevenly acquainted with the truth. Not divided, not polarized — simply uneven. In every audience, no matter the continent or the discipline represented, there were people encountering the molecular relationship for the very first time. Their faces revealed it instantly: not skepticism, but a kind of startled recalibration, the quiet realization that a gap in their understanding had just been illuminated.

He never resented this. In fact, he expected it.

The old warnings had been broadcast for so long, and with such moral urgency, that entire generations of clinicians and researchers had internalized them without ever encountering the underlying biochemistry. People weren’t resisting him — they had simply inherited a narrative without knowing its origins.

What moved him most was how similar the reaction looked across cultures.

Whether he was speaking in Reykjavik or Seoul, in a London hall filled with clinical advisors or a modest symposium in the Midwest, the moment of first comprehension had the same quiet shape. A slight tilt of the head. A softening of the brow. A long pause before the next note was taken. No alarm, no defensiveness — simply recognition that something essential had been overlooked in the rush to protect.

He learned to guide that recognition gently.

Not by overwhelming listeners with data, but by offering the science with calm proportion, allowing the molecular architecture to reveal itself at its own pace. He knew that too forceful an approach could trigger resistance in people who were already balancing multiple responsibilities. So he introduced the concept the way morning light enters a room — gradually, illuminating only what needs to be seen first.

And always, after these presentations, there was a moment — sometimes brief, sometimes lingering — when an attendee approached him privately. Their tone was never confrontational; it was reflective, as though they were piecing together the implications in real time.

“I had no idea selenium played such a role.”

“Why wasn’t this emphasized in training?”

“How did we miss this for so long?”

Or the simplest, said with a kind of humbled honesty:

“This changes things.”

He never responded with triumph.

He responded with proportion.

“The science has been steady all along,” he would say. “Sometimes the narrative takes longer to catch up.”

He said it not as an indictment, but as a reassurance. Because he understood that the slowness of the correction was not a failure of intelligence — it was a consequence of momentum. Fear moves quickly; clarity moves with deliberation. And the old guidance had been fear-based, even if issued with good intentions.

He often found himself reflecting on this dynamic during the quiet moments after a talk — sitting alone in a hotel room overlooking a foreign city, or walking back to his lodging through narrow streets lit by late evening lamps. He would think about how unevenly truth spreads, how some minds absorb it instantly while others require years of exposure. He never judged the disparity. He simply noted it with the same observational steadiness he brought to the laboratory.

What mattered wasn't how many people understood him on any given day.

What mattered was that the understanding was spreading — quietly, proportionately, in widening circles of influence. A clinician here. A researcher there. A policymaker who heard something new and carried it home. The correction did not travel evenly, but it traveled faithfully. And faithfulness, he knew, was more powerful than speed.

In these reflections, he felt neither loneliness nor urgency — only continuity.

His work had entered a phase where truth moved not because he pushed, but because it resonated. The world was still catching up, but it was catching up honestly, without theatrics, without resistance, one mind at a time.

He carried that knowledge with him as he traveled home, settling into his seat on the plane with the calm understanding that influence does not require universality. It requires durability. And the truth he carried — quiet, molecular, protective — was proving itself durable.

There were flights home when he pressed his forehead lightly against the cool window and watched the lights of a foreign city recede beneath him, shrinking into a latticework of distant glimmers. These departures always carried the same feeling — not closure, not fatigue, but a quiet accounting. He would replay the conversations of the previous days in his mind, not to measure their success, but to understand the subtle shifts that had occurred.

He had learned something over the years:

the most important transformations in a field rarely announced themselves in applause or headlines.

They showed themselves in tone.

A question asked with curiosity rather than caution.

A colleague lingering after a session, not to debate but to clarify.

An advisory board member approaching him with the quiet admission that they had never considered the implications of proportionality before.

These moments were small, but they were directional.

They pointed toward a world slowly relinquishing its attachment to an outdated warning.

He often thought about how strange it was that the slowness of the correction had become one of the clearest signals of its legitimacy. Fast shifts in public health usually indicated fashion, panic, or political pressure. But this shift — the recognition of selenium's protective role — was moving with the deliberate cadence of something real. Something earned. Something that had survived decades of scrutiny and still remained intact.

He felt this most clearly during a symposium in Northern Europe where, after he finished speaking, an older epidemiologist approached him. Her expression held neither skepticism nor urgency — only contemplation.

"I think we were too ready to treat the uncertainty as danger," she said quietly. "And too slow to treat the data as guidance."

He nodded gently, because the sentence carried no blame. It carried a truth he had lived for most of his professional life. She looked down at her notes, then added, almost to herself, "We built a warning before we understood the context."

He had no corrective to offer.

She had already corrected herself.

In moments like that, he realized that the world did not need to be convinced — it needed to be reminded. Reminded that science evolves. Reminded that balance matters. Reminded that fear, once institutionalized, can persist long after its justification has weakened. And reminded that the developing brain deserved not panic, but clarity.

He carried these reflections with him as the plane leveled off above the cloud line. The cabin dimmed to its soft, blue-grey light. People settled into silence. He found himself thinking of the unborn children whose mothers had avoided fish out of misunderstood caution

— children who might have gone without essential nutrients because the narrative had been too loud, too confident, and too incomplete.

He never dwelled on regret.

But he understood responsibility.

Responsibility to ensure that the future mothers of the world would not inherit the same distortion. Responsibility to ensure that clinicians would not continue to repeat warnings born of old assumptions. Responsibility to ensure that the truth was no longer the domain of conferences alone, but the quiet knowledge of every practitioner who advised someone carrying a new life.

He closed his eyes for a moment, feeling the steady vibration of the engines, the familiar hum of altitude. In that stillness, he sensed the arc of his work as though it were a constellation — a pattern only visible from a distance, shaped by years of persistence, patience, and restraint.

The world had not yet fully arrived at the correction.

But it was unmistakably moving toward it.

And he would continue to guide that movement the only way he knew how — gently, proportionately, without spectacle — until the truth no longer needed his voice to be understood.

There were seasons — long, unremarkable, quietly accumulative seasons — when the work advanced not through new discoveries, but through the gradual softening of the world's certainty. He came to understand that certainty was the true barrier, not ignorance. Ignorance was flexible. Certainty was rigid.

And the old warnings, repeated for decades with a kind of moral confidence, had hardened into a certainty that lived not in data, but in instinct.

This was why change moved slowly.

Not because the science was complicated.

But because people mistook repetition for truth.

He thought about this often during his walks across campus, especially in late spring when the river finally freed itself from ice and the wind carried the scent of thawed soil. The path that ran alongside the water had become a place for reflection, a kind of private observatory where he could consider the strange, quiet persistence of the old narrative.

It struck him as almost poetic:

that a misunderstanding could survive simply because it had once been convenient.

Convenient for advisory boards.

Convenient for policymakers.

Convenient for organizations that preferred simple warnings over nuanced truths.

Fear, after all, was easy to teach.

Proportion was not.

And yet, despite the inertia of certainty, he could feel the gradual erosion occurring. Not in dramatic gestures, but in subtle shifts of language. Words that once carried absolute weight — "danger," "avoid," "toxic" — were being replaced with more careful phrasing. Phrases like "balance," "context," "nutrient interaction." The world had begun to speak more softly. Softness, he knew, was the early sign of correction.

One afternoon, during a meeting with a regional health consortium, he noticed this linguistic shift in real time. A nutrition director, flipping through her notes, paused and said, almost offhandedly, "Of course, we also have to consider the biochemical context when we talk about fetal development."

She didn't look up. She didn't emphasize the phrase. She didn't seem to realize she had spoken a sentence that would have been unimaginable twenty years ago.

He felt the weight of that moment all the same.

The correction had begun to live inside ordinary language.

Later that week, while preparing data for a lecture, he found himself revisiting an early paper he had written at a time when the field was deeply entrenched in its caution-first posture. He remembered every frustration that had accompanied it — the reviews that asked him to "soften the implications," the colleagues who advised him to "choose a different hill," the institutional reluctance to incorporate anything that challenged the comfortable warnings.

Reading it now, he felt no resentment.

Only perspective.

He saw a younger version of himself standing at the edge of a landscape that had not yet shifted, holding a truth that few were ready to hear. It was strange to revisit that moment knowing what came after — the slow diffusion of understanding, the incremental acceptance, the steady rewiring of the world's nutritional instincts. He realized that everything he had done in those early years had been an act of faith, even if he never thought of it that way at the time.

Faith not in himself, but in proportion.

Faith in balance.

Faith in the inherent integrity of the molecules.

He set the old paper aside and allowed himself a brief, reflective breath. The world was not yet fully aligned with the correction — but it was unmistakably closer. The old certainty had begun to crack, replaced not by a new certainty but by a more honest posture: humility.

Humility, he thought, was the real victory.

Not that the world agreed with him,

but that the world had learned to reconsider.

That reconsideration, small as it seemed, was the single most important change in the entire landscape. It meant the next generation of researchers would not inherit the rigidity that had slowed progress for so long. It meant future clinicians would speak to pregnant mothers with clarity instead of inherited fear. It meant the misunderstanding would eventually fade — not by force, but by irrelevance.

He sat back in his chair as the late afternoon light stretched across his desk, and he felt the steady, grounded satisfaction of someone watching the world finally tilt, even if by degrees, toward the right direction.

The correction was no longer a hope.

It was a progression.

A slow one, yes.

But slow things, he had learned, endure.

There were mid-summer days when the science building felt almost deserted, the hallways carrying only the faint hum of ventilation and the distant echo of someone's footsteps a floor above. He had always liked the building best in these quiet months. Without the traffic of students or the pace of faculty meetings, the place felt more like a sanctuary than an institution — a space where thought could stretch without interruption.

He often spent these days reviewing correspondence from organizations around the world. Some letters came from major public health agencies, others from quiet local practitioners who had stumbled onto his work after exhausting all other explanations. The tone of these messages varied widely, but each carried its own small truth about where the correction currently lived.

Some writers spoke with a conviction that suggested they had been waiting years for someone to articulate what they already sensed.

Others wrote with the cautious curiosity of people beginning to loosen their grip on an old belief.

And some wrote with a kind of weary honesty — acknowledging that they did not know how the narrative had gone so wrong for so long, but determined not to let error persist beyond their own tenure.

He read each message with the same steady attention, never rushing through them, never treating any of them as routine. The diversity of voices reminded him that truth spreads not through consensus, but through sincerity. A single clinician in a small town could shift more real-world outcomes than an entire board of advisors who moved too slowly.

It was during one of these quiet summer afternoons that he received a letter from a midwife in coastal New England. She wrote not from a place of theory, but from lived experience. For twenty years, she had unintentionally discouraged mothers from eating fish out of fear. Recently, after encountering his research, she had reconsidered her practice. She now encouraged fish consumption, explained the protective balance, and monitored outcomes with a discerning eye.

"I can't undo the years," she wrote.

"But I can correct the years ahead."

He sat with that sentence for a long moment.

It was the purest distillation of everything he had hoped for — not perfection, not repentance, not spectacle — just a shift in posture. A willingness to realign. A quiet redirection of influence. The kind of correction that begins in a single room with a single voice and radiates outward in ways no data model could ever predict.

He found himself thinking about all the unseen rooms where the truth now lived.

Clinics.

Classrooms.

Nutrition counseling sessions.

Community workshops.

Medical trainings.

Places where he would never set foot — yet where the molecular reality he had carried for decades had begun to reshape decisions, conversations, instincts.

Influence, he realized, was not measured by recognition.

Influence was measured by continuity.

The next day, during a lecture in a small auditorium, he felt that continuity in real time. The attendees were not prestigious researchers or policy directors. They were local healthcare workers — nurses, midwives, wellness counselors. People who dealt with the lived realities of pregnancy rather than the abstractions of policy.

He explained the relationship gently, weaving the biochemistry with the clarity of someone who had spent a lifetime translating complexity into coherence. As he spoke, he noticed how many in the room nodded slowly — not because they had known the science, but because the science matched something they had observed in their own practices without having the vocabulary to explain it.

This was always his favorite reaction:

the recognition that arrives before understanding.

The sense that the truth had been waiting for its name.

After the talk, a young nurse approached him. She held a notebook filled with quick, handwritten observations.

"I never knew why fish mattered so much," she said. "I mean, I knew it was important, but I didn't know why. You just made it make sense."

He smiled, not out of pride, but out of a kind of quiet relief — relief that clarity had reached another room, another mind, another future mother.

Walking back across campus afterward, he felt the familiar calm of someone who understands that his work no longer travels only through conferences or journals. It travels through conversations. Through explanations given in exam rooms. Through the moment a clinician pauses before repeating an old warning and instead chooses a new truth.

Corrective work, he thought, is never swift.

But once it begins to move through lived practice, it becomes irreversible.

The late afternoon sun stretched long bands of gold across the concrete walkway, warming the air in a way that felt almost ceremonial. He paused at the top of the steps, looking out across the quiet campus, and let the moment settle.

The alignment was spreading.

Not evenly, not loudly, but faithfully.

Exactly as it should.

There were autumn weeks when the trees on campus turned a deep, burnished gold, and he felt an odd symmetry between the landscape and the work. The leaves shifted slowly at first, almost imperceptibly, then all at once the branches carried a new color, a new clarity, a new truth. He often thought that change in public health followed the same rhythm — invisible at the beginning, undeniable in retrospect.

He walked these paths deliberately, observing the subtle transitions in tone around him. Conversations had changed. Lectures had changed. Even the questions students asked had changed. Not dramatically — nothing about this work ever moved dramatically — but steadily, like a tide advancing grain by grain.

In one of his graduate seminars, he posed a question about nutrient interactions, expecting the discussion to unfold the way it always had. But a young student — soft-spoken, precise — raised her hand and said something that stopped him.

"Isn't the real issue how fear shaped the guidance more than the molecules did?"

He felt the room shift.

Not because the observation was revolutionary, but because it was articulated without hesitation. Without defensiveness. Without the inherited reverence for the old warnings that had lingered for so long. Her tone carried a kind of clean, intellectual honesty — the kind that suggested she had not grown up inside the distortion and therefore did not feel obligated to defend it.

It struck him that this was the first generation of students being trained without the reflexive fear that had once permeated the field. They were learning biochemistry before bureaucracy. Proportion before panic. And in them, he sensed the beginning of something he had waited decades to see: a generation for whom the correction was not controversial, but intuitive.

After class, he lingered by the window overlooking the campus green. Leaves drifted down in slow spirals, catching the late light. He realized that the shift had become self-sustaining. Even if he retired tomorrow, the truth would continue to propagate through these students, through their future practices, through the mothers and children whose lives would be shaped by their advice.

The work no longer depended on him.

It lived independently now — diffused, distributed, embodied by others.

He returned to his office with this understanding settling over him like a quiet mantle. He sat down, opened a folder of recent correspondence, and found a letter from a national nutrition council he had once assumed would never revise its position. Their tone had changed. They requested updated explanations, updated phrasing, updated considerations.

There was no apology — he had never expected one.

There was simply recalibration.

Recalibration was the closest thing institutions ever offered to contrition.

He drafted a response with the same calm precision that defined the rest of his work. He did not rush. He did not overstate. He simply offered the truth in its most coherent form — the same truth he had been offering since the beginning.

As he typed, he felt a curious stillness rise within him — not satisfaction, but alignment. Alignment between decades of effort and the world's slow willingness to see what should have been evident all along. He thought of all the unborn children who would benefit from future guidance shaped by clarity rather than fear, and for the first time, he allowed himself to feel the magnitude of that impact.

He closed his laptop gently, folded his hands, and stared for a moment at the fading light outside his window. The corridor of his career — long, quiet, sometimes lonely — had finally begun to open. There was still work to do, yes, but the resistance had softened. The world had begun to listen with a different posture.

Truth, he realized, had its own seasons.

And this season belonged to proportion.

He rose from his chair, turned off the light, and stepped into the hallway, feeling the quiet dignity of someone who has carried a truth long enough for the world to finally catch up.

There were early winter mornings when the frost along the laboratory windows formed intricate, crystalline patterns — delicate, branching geometries that mimicked the complexity of the molecules he had spent his life studying. He often paused at the glass before turning on the lights, drawn not to the cold or the view outside, but to the strange comfort he found in these fleeting shapes. They reminded him of something essential: that even temporary structures could reveal enduring truths.

The world, he thought, often confused permanence with significance.

But significance was rarely permanent at first.

It emerged in increments, through small corrections, through patterns that appeared briefly and then reappeared again later in more stable forms.

He saw this happening everywhere now.

One morning, he opened a journal and found an editorial — not a study, not a breakthrough, but an editorial — discussing the role of nutrient balance in fetal development. It was cautious, written with the politeness of an institution that understood it was revising a long-standing posture without wanting to announce the revision too loudly. But the shift was unmistakable. The language had begun to change.

Not wholesale.

Not boldly.

But unmistakably.

Phrases that had once been unthinkable had slipped into the text:

"emerging clarity"

"proportional understanding"

"contextual risk"

"protective interaction"

These were not his phrases. He had never insisted on a lexicon. But they carried the fingerprints of the correction. Not because anyone had quoted him, but because the science itself had become impossible to ignore.

He closed the journal and let the quiet settle.

It was a different kind of satisfaction — not personal, not triumphant — but structural. The kind of satisfaction a bridge engineer might feel decades after construction, seeing that the foundation had held through weather, bureaucracy, and the slow erosion of misconceptions.

Later that week, he was invited to give a guest lecture to a cohort of graduate students who were preparing to enter clinical practice. The lecture hall was modest, the seating slightly uneven, the projector humming faintly as he adjusted the slides. He had delivered versions of this talk for years, but something about the room felt different before he even began.

The students were attentive in a way that suggested they had already shifted beyond the old narrative. Their questions weren't defensive; they were exploratory. They weren't grappling with fear; they were grappling with nuance. They weren't inheriting the past; they were constructing the future.

Halfway through the session, a student seated near the front raised her hand and asked a question that struck him with its simplicity:

"If the biochemistry is this clear, why did the world get stuck on the wrong idea for so long?"

He considered the question carefully — not because he didn't know the answer, but because he wanted to honor the honesty behind it. He had asked himself the same thing countless times over the years, in hallways, in meetings, in solitude.

"Because fear is easier to communicate than balance," he said softly. "And once a fear takes hold, it begins to feel like duty."

She nodded slowly, understanding not just the explanation but the history folded within it.

After the lecture, he lingered as students gathered their notebooks and laptops. One paused at the door, turned back, and said, “I’m glad we’re learning this now. Earlier would have been better, but now is something.”

He watched her leave, and a realization settled over him like a layer of newly fallen snow:

the next generation would not repeat the mistake.

They would not inherit fear unexamined.

They would not perpetuate warnings without context.

They would treat proportion not as a footnote, but as a foundation.

The old narrative was dissolving — not dramatically, but steadily. It was being replaced not by his voice, but by their understanding. That shift, he knew, would have a greater impact on the world than anything he could publish.

Walking back across campus, he noticed the first thin ice forming along the edges of the river. It was delicate at this stage, fragile, almost transparent. But he knew how these things worked. The edges strengthened first. The center followed. Change always began at the periphery, then advanced inward with quiet certainty.

The correction was following the same physics.

Strengthening at the edges.

Advancing toward the center.

Becoming inevitable.

He turned his collar up against the wind and continued toward the science building, carrying with him the calm, steady conviction of someone who could finally see the long arc of the work — not behind him, but moving ahead on its own momentum.

There were evenings when he stayed late not out of obligation, but out of a quiet instinct — the sense that something in the world was shifting again, almost imperceptibly, and he wanted to be present for it. The building settled around him in a way that only older academic structures can, with soft clicks in the radiators and a faint, continuous hum from equipment left running overnight. He liked the building best in these hours. It felt honest then, stripped of ceremony, stripped of performance. Just a place where truth had been worked on for decades, grain by grain.

He sat at his desk reviewing a set of international guidelines recently released by a consortium he had long assumed would be among the last to update their stance. He didn't expect much — perhaps a softened phrase, perhaps a footnote acknowledging complexity — but as he read, he felt a quiet stirring, even before he reached the section on maternal seafood consumption.

The language had changed.

Not dramatically. Not even boldly. But unmistakably.

Where there had once been categorical warnings, there was now cautious nuance.

Where there had once been prohibitions, there were now contextual considerations.

Where there had once been the unmistakable tone of fear, there was now something closer to humility.

He read the paragraph again, slower this time.

He could almost pinpoint the sentences where an old assumption had been reluctantly surrendered.

He could feel the internal debate behind each softened clause.

He closed the document and let the stillness settle over him.

This was how change looked in institutions — not like a declaration, but like erosion. The kind of erosion that takes years, then suddenly becomes visible all at once. You never see the individual grains fall away. You only see the new shape when you step back.

He leaned back in his chair, hands folded loosely, and thought about all the nights he had spent in this same room years earlier — nights when he reviewed data no one wanted to hear, when he practiced lectures that would be met with polite resistance, when he drafted papers that would be accepted only after reviewers had softened the language to make the truth less disruptive.

To sit here now, reading guidelines that finally approached clarity, felt strangely unspectacular — and that was exactly right. Corrections, when they finally arrive, should feel natural, not dramatic.

He turned off the lamp and made his way down the hallway. The motion-sensor lights flickered on ahead of him, illuminating the corridor in soft increments. He paused at the window halfway down and looked out over the quiet campus. Snow had begun falling — small flakes at first, drifting without urgency, settling onto the branches and pathways with silent intention.

Snow always reminded him of the work:

accumulative, quiet, indifferent to resistance, altering the landscape without needing anyone's permission.

As he stood there, he thought of all the people he had met over the years who had been caught between inherited fear and emerging clarity — clinicians torn between duty and doubt, researchers who sensed the imbalance but lacked the vocabulary to confront it, policymakers overwhelmed by the tension between protecting the public and updating the narrative responsibly.

Now, slowly, the tension was dissolving.

Not because the old warnings had been disproven in one moment, but because the new understanding had proved itself across decades.

He made his way to the exit and stepped outside, pulling his coat a little tighter. The snow had begun falling more steadily now, softening the sounds of the night. The air was sharp, clean, and almost meditative. He walked toward the parking lot, hearing the crunch of fresh snowfall under his boots, and felt the unmistakable calm of alignment — the kind that appears only after years of work have finally begun to match the world's awareness.

As he reached his car, he paused once more to look across the snowy campus, its lights glowing faintly through the drift.

He realized that the work no longer needed urgency.

It no longer needed defense.

It no longer needed explanation delivered with extra care.

It simply needed time — and time, at long last, was cooperating.

He brushed the snow from the door handle, opened it, and settled into the seat. The silence inside the car felt warm compared to the cold outside, a small pocket of stillness at the edge of a long, measured journey.

He exhaled slowly, watching the breath fade into the air before him.

The correction was no longer fragile.

It had entered its lasting phase.

There were late-winter conferences held in cities where the cold seemed to arrive from every direction at once — through the wind, through the architecture, even through the language. He often found himself walking between venues bundled tightly against the elements, the air so sharp it seemed to clarify his thoughts simply by passing through them. These trips were part of the rhythm of his year, and although the locations differed, the atmosphere inside the buildings was always the same: warm, earnest, slightly overstated in its decor, with lanyards and paper programs that all carried the same aesthetic of institutional confidence.

But what he found inside those rooms had begun to change.

Not the decor, not the formalities, not the choreography of keynote speakers and panel discussions. What had changed was subtler — a new texture in the questions, a new honesty in the pauses, a new softness in the posture of people who had, for too long, armored themselves in inherited certainty.

On one such evening, after delivering his session to a room of public health practitioners, he attended the post-conference reception — an event he usually drifted through quietly, taking in the atmosphere without expecting much. But this time, something different happened. Not dramatic, not loud, not even particularly emotional. Just... different.

A physician approached him with a glass of something sparkling, her badge half-turned on its lanyard, the expression on her face that of someone who had been carrying a question for a long time and had finally found the person to ask.

"I've been practicing for 18 years," she began. "During all that time, we were trained to lead with caution. To simplify the message. To remove nuance because we thought patients needed certainty. And I'm realizing now that certainty is what misled us."

He watched her carefully — not to judge, but to understand the shape of her admission. She wasn't apologizing. She wasn't excusing. She was doing something far more important: she was acknowledging the interior cost of inheriting a narrative that turned out to be incomplete.

She continued, softer now.

"When you showed that the guidance didn't account for the biochemical interaction... it wasn't just the science that hit me. It was the responsibility. I've spent years counseling pregnant women away from fish. I thought I was protecting them."

He knew better than to fill the silence too quickly. Overcorrection helped no one. Clarity required space.

"You were acting on the knowledge available to you," he said finally, his voice low and steady. "And now you're acting on better knowledge. That is what science is supposed to be."

She nodded, but the nod held something deeper than agreement — it held release. As though a weight she hadn't quite recognized had finally loosened its hold.

Moments like this, he realized, were the true markers of progress: not the publications, not the policy drafts, not the quiet edits slipping into institutional guidelines. But the individual reckonings. The quiet recalibrations in the minds of people whose daily work touched real lives.

He left the reception early, stepping into the crisp night air. Snowflakes drifted down in slow spirals, catching the lamplight as though suspended in thought. He walked back to his hotel without haste, listening to the muffled sound of his footsteps against the fresh accumulation.

Along the way, he thought about all the unseen consequences of the old warnings — the meals avoided, the nutrients missed, the decisions shaped by fear rather than proportion. He did not linger on these thoughts out of regret, but out of commitment. He understood that correcting a narrative required as much patience as the narrative had taken to form.

When he reached the hotel lobby, he paused for a moment near the entrance, watching other attendees return from the reception — some in animated conversation, others quietly absorbed. A few glanced at him with the expression he had come to recognize:

respect mixed with a kind of dawning awareness. They would carry the correction forward in their own ways, through conversations with colleagues, through revised patient guidance, through the private shift in how they spoke about risk.

He took the elevator to his room and sat for a while in the quiet, looking out at the city through a window that framed the falling snow like a slow-moving veil.

He realized something then — something that felt both simple and profound:

The work had entered a new phase.

No longer a debate.

No longer a defense.

Just a slow, steady unfolding of clarity.

A kind of intellectual thaw.

The world wasn't rushing toward the truth.

It was warming toward it.

And that warmth — subtle, cumulative, persistent — would do more for the next generation than any argument ever could.

He closed the curtains gently, letting the room return to its soft interior light, and prepared for the next day with the steady assurance of someone who understood that the correction was now inevitable not because he insisted, but because the world had begun to understand itself more clearly.

There were stretches of early spring when the world outside the laboratory felt strangely unsettled — not in a disruptive way, but in the way a landscape feels when something long frozen begins, silently, to loosen. He noticed it first in the river. A hairline crack would appear one morning along the ice, faint as a whisper. The next day, it would widen by half an inch. Then, without warning, a long sheet of ice would detach from the shoreline and drift, slow and deliberate, toward the center.

He had always liked this stage of the thaw.

Not the dramatic break.

Not the loud cracking that made headlines.

But the quiet transitions — the ones that signaled inevitability.

The correction he had spent his life stewarding was entering that same stage.

He could sense it in places he never expected — in the questions people no longer asked, in the assumptions that no longer held authority, in the vocabulary that no longer sounded natural. The world had not reversed itself. It had simply lost interest in defending a mistake.

Progress often arrived disguised as disinterest.

One afternoon, he attended a virtual roundtable hosted by a coalition of maternal health researchers. It was informal, the sort of gathering where people spoke candidly because no one was taking minutes. He listened quietly as they discussed new approaches to patient counseling, the impact of emerging nutrient data, and the revision of outdated communication strategies.

At one point, a clinician said, almost casually, “I think we’re done frightening people about fish. It never aligned with the evidence.”

There was no debate. No pushback. No need for him to intervene.

The sentence simply drifted across the group, settled, and was accepted — as though it had always been obvious.

He turned his camera off for a moment, not out of frustration or fatigue, but out of something closer to contemplation. He realized that he had waited decades to hear that kind of sentence spoken without ceremony. The world had finally reached a point where clarity no longer required advocacy — it required only recognition.

After the meeting ended, he walked across campus, following the same path he had walked thousands of times. Students hurried by in light jackets, their conversations filled with the easy optimism of early spring. The air held the faint scent of thawed earth — a smell that carried its own kind of promise.

He stopped on the pedestrian bridge and leaned on the railing, watching the river move beneath him. The ice had broken apart into long, drifting segments, each piece reflecting a softened version of the grey-blue sky. The movement was slow, almost ceremonial, as though the river were rediscovering its own freedom molecule by molecule.

For years, he had felt a parallel sense of confinement — not physical, but conceptual. The old warnings had acted like ice, holding the narrative in place long after the current beneath had shifted. Now, finally, the surface had begun to break. The river and the work seemed to be unfolding in the same cadence, each revealing what had always been true beneath the frozen gloss.

As he stood there, he found himself thinking not of the conferences or the journals or the policy papers, but of the children — the children whose lives would be shaped by decisions their mothers made long before birth. The children who needed clarity, not cautionary folklore. The children for whom the world would now be a little more proportionate, a little more honest, a little more aligned with what nature intended.

He watched a long pane of ice tilt, catch the current, and slip downstream.

Change, he realized, did not require applause.

It required persistence.

And persistence, once it reaches a certain threshold, becomes irreversible.

He remained on the bridge a few minutes longer, letting the breeze carry away the last remnants of winter air. Then he turned and made his way back toward the science building, walking with the steady, unhurried stride of someone who understood the new landscape — not perfectly, but deeply.

The thaw had begun.

And the thaw, unlike the freeze, never asked permission.

There were afternoons in late spring when the science building filled with a soft, almost weightless light — the kind that entered through high windows and diffused across the linoleum floors like a slow-moving tide. He always noticed how different the building felt in this season. The corridors, usually colored by winter's austerity, seemed warmer, more forgiving, as though the place itself was exhaling after months of muted cold.

On one such afternoon, he found himself walking toward a small departmental gathering — an informal seminar series intended to give researchers a chance to share updates without the pressure of formal presentations. He had attended these for years, often as a quiet observer, sometimes as a speaker. Today, he planned simply to listen.

He took a seat near the back of the room, notebook closed, hands folded loosely. The seminar began with a brief overview of recent projects — nutrient studies, public health surveys, environmental assessments. But about halfway through, something unexpected happened. A young researcher, perhaps early in her career, stood at the front of the room and spoke about the challenges of communicating complex scientific truths to the public.

Without referencing him directly, without drawing attention to any controversy, she said something that caught his full attention.

"We made a mistake," she said plainly, "when we believed that oversimplifying the message would protect people. It didn't. It limited them."

The room shifted.

Not in shock — in agreement.

She continued, her tone steadier than her years might have suggested.

“We told pregnant women to fear the wrong thing. And in doing so, we prevented them from accessing nutrients essential for their children’s development. We need to replace fear with proportion, because proportion aligns with biology.”

He recognized the phrasing, the cadence, the underlying principle — not because she was quoting him, but because she was speaking from a place shaped by the new landscape he had helped form.

It was an extraordinary thing to witness:

someone articulating a truth he had carried for decades

as if it were simply the way things were.

Not revolutionary.

Not controversial.

Just... correct.

He felt no impulse to speak. He didn’t raise his hand. He didn’t offer commentary during the question period. He simply sat there, letting the moment unfold, letting its quiet significance take shape.

After the seminar ended, he lingered in the hallway as people mingled. A few nodded at him in passing — the polite, understated recognition colleagues often exchange in academic spaces. But no one approached him with urgency. No one asked him to defend the work. No one treated him as a figure standing on the frontier of a debate.

And that — strangely, beautifully — was the clearest sign of progress.

The frontier had moved.

Not because he pushed it,

but because the world had finally begun to walk toward it on its own.

He left the gathering and stepped outside into the late afternoon light. The air was mild, the wind soft, carrying hints of early summer. Students sprawled across the grass in loose circles, their textbooks scattered around them like the debris of optimism. He walked slowly, allowing the warmth to settle into his shoulders.

Along the walkway, he passed a young couple — presumably students — discussing prenatal nutrition for a project. He caught only a fragment of their conversation:

"...the important thing is balance, not avoidance..."

That was enough.

Two students, chatting casually, repeating something that had once been treated as dangerous truth.

He continued walking, scarcely altering his pace.

He thought about how the correction had seeped into the culture — not through mandates or controversies, but through steady dissemination. It now existed in the informal spaces: classrooms, study groups, quiet conversations on campus greens. It was no longer dependent on his advocacy. It had become part of the shared intellectual atmosphere.

As he approached the science building once more, he paused to look at its façade — a structure he had walked into thousands of times, each time carrying some fragment of truth he hoped the world would eventually see.

Now, standing there in the warm light, he felt something rare and immeasurable:

a sense of proximity between the world as it was and the world as it could be.

The work was not finished.

But it was no longer alone.

He walked up the steps slowly, not out of fatigue, but out of awareness — the kind of awareness that comes from seeing a long arc bend, not all at once, but undeniably, toward clarity.

Inside, the building greeted him with its familiar quiet, and he felt the calm certainty of someone who knows the next movement will unfold exactly as it should.

There were evenings in early summer when the campus seemed suspended in a kind of gentle equilibrium — the sun lingering longer than expected, the air warm but not yet heavy, the sky still carrying the faintest memory of winter's clarity. He often walked during these hours, not out of routine, but out of instinct. The quiet suited him. The soft light suited the work. And the transitional season — neither fully one thing nor the other — echoed the moment he found himself in professionally.

The world was no longer resisting the correction.

But it had not yet fully embraced it.

It lived in the in-between, which was precisely where truth often matured.

One evening, as he crossed the broad lawn behind the science building, he noticed an outdoor public health workshop taking place beneath a cluster of elm trees. A few folding tables had been set up, brochures neatly stacked in small piles, and a young instructor was speaking to a circle of expectant mothers. He slowed his pace, careful not to draw attention, and simply observed from a respectful distance.

He expected the usual talking points — hydration, folate, iron, sleep hygiene. But as he listened, he realized something had shifted. The instructor spoke with a calm balance, neither sensational nor overly cautious. When she reached the topic of nutrition, she said something that stopped him in his tracks.

"Ocean fish are one of the best foods you can eat," she said. "They contain natural protection that supports fetal development."

No fear.

No qualifiers.

No inherited warnings.

Just clarity — simple, direct, unburdened.

One of the mothers raised her hand hesitantly. "I thought we were supposed to avoid fish? Something about mercury?"

The instructor smiled gently, not dismissively but with the confidence of someone who understood the science rather than the folklore.

"That was the old thinking," she said. "We've learned more since then. The nutrients in fish protect the developing brain. The balance matters more than the fear."

He felt the air shift inside him, a slow, inward settling.

This was not a conference.

Not a peer-reviewed journal.

Not a policy meeting or an advisory panel.

This was where the real work lived — in the open air, on a mild evening, spoken calmly to those whose lives would be most directly shaped by the truth.

He stood there for a moment longer than he intended, then continued walking. But something stayed with him — the phrase the instructor had used, almost casually:

"That was the old thinking."

It occurred to him that he had waited most of his life to hear someone speak that sentence aloud without defensiveness. It was the sound of a mistake dissolving. The sound of a narrative relinquishing its hold. The sound of fear losing its claim to authority.

Later that night, sitting on a bench overlooking the river, he watched the lights of downtown shimmer on the water. The current flowed with a calm steadiness, carrying reflections downstream in long, wavering ribbons. He realized that the correction had reached a point where it could no longer be reversed. Not because of any single publication or lecture, but because it had entered the lexicon of everyday care.

Once a truth enters the world through ordinary voices, it becomes permanent.

He leaned back, feeling the subtle warmth radiating from the bench's wooden slats, and allowed the quiet to settle around him. In the distance, he could hear students laughing, a dog barking near the footpath, the faint thrum of a bicycle passing behind him. Life unfolding, unconcerned with the long arc of scientific correction.

But he knew better.

He understood that these ordinary sounds belonged to the same world that would benefit from the change — the world that would eventually raise children whose mothers had been advised with precision rather than imprecision, with proportion rather than panic.

The correction was no longer an argument.

It was a fact.

A fact spoken to mothers beneath elm trees on warm evenings.

A fact carried into clinics by young clinicians who had never known the old warnings.

A fact whispered across generations without anyone needing to remember when the shift occurred.

He closed his eyes, letting the evening breeze move gently across his face.

It had taken decades.

It had required patience few would have had the stamina to maintain.

But the long corridor had finally begun to open at both ends — past and future, meeting in the present with the quiet elegance of alignment.

He opened his eyes slowly and stood, the night deepening around him.

There were late-summer mornings when the world felt almost too quiet — as though the day itself were pausing before deciding what posture to take. He often arrived at the lab early on such mornings, long before the hallways filled, long before the sounds of printers and conversations and scheduled obligations reasserted themselves. The building, in that early hush, felt like a companion rather than a workplace.

He would unlock the door, step into his office, and stand for a moment without turning on the lights. The ambient glow from the hallway was enough. In that dim, transitional light he could feel the entire arc of the work — past and future braided together in a single, almost imperceptible thread.

It was on one such morning that he opened his email and found a message from a former student — now a pediatrician working in a rural region far from any academic center. She wrote with a tone he recognized instantly: calm, certain, unhurried. She described a patient — a young expectant mother who had arrived fearful, overwhelmed by conflicting advice she had gathered from the internet, family, and outdated pamphlets at her local clinic.

"I explained the balance," the doctor wrote. "I explained what the nutrients actually do, what the body actually needs. And for the first time in her pregnancy, she relaxed. She said no one had ever told her the truth so plainly."

He read the line twice.

It wasn't the praise that struck him — she had not intended praise — but the word plainly. The truth had finally become plain enough to guide someone else's clarity without requiring him in the room.

He sat back in his chair, letting the realization drift in.

For decades, the truth had been anything but plain.

It had been obscured by institutional caution, diluted by misunderstanding, and burdened by the weight of inherited fear. He had spent years untangling narratives, years defending proportions, years explaining what should have been obvious: that the body protects life with remarkable intelligence, and that the molecules themselves explained more than the warnings ever had.

Now, here was a physician — once a student in the back row of his seminar — carrying that truth forward with steadiness, without hesitation, without needing to borrow his voice.

He responded briefly, not out of modesty but out of recognition:

"You did the real work. You offered clarity."

After sending the message, he set his laptop aside and walked to the window. Outside, the trees were still lush, but the edges of some leaves had begun to pale — the faintest whisper of the approaching shift. The light carried that same transitional quality, neither the bright assertiveness of midsummer nor the softened melancholy of autumn.

He felt something inside him echoing that shift.

For years, he had carried the correction like a private burden — a responsibility born not of ego but of precision. He had lived with the knowledge that the world's fear-directed guidance was not only incorrect, but quietly harmful. He had shouldered that discrepancy without bitterness, using patience instead of force, using proportion instead of confrontation.

Now, slowly, the burden was redistributing itself.

Clarified thinking was taking root in places he would never see.

The truth he had once protected was beginning to protect itself.

Later that afternoon, he attended a small committee meeting on campus — the type of meeting he had learned long ago required more listening than speaking. As he took his seat at the long wooden table, he noticed something different in the room before anyone spoke.

Not excitement.

Not urgency.

Something quieter.

A posture of consideration.

The chair opened with a brief overview of updated educational materials being drafted for community clinics. Someone mentioned the need to revise outdated sections on maternal seafood consumption. Then another committee member — someone he would not have predicted years earlier — spoke up.

"We should make sure the new materials reflect the current science," she said. "We owe women accuracy, not echoes."

He didn't move.

Didn't nod.

Didn't smile.

But inside, a quiet recognition unfolded — a recognition that the language had changed even before the policies had. The shift was happening in thought, in instinct, in unguarded sentences uttered in modest committee rooms.

He contributed when asked — precise, concise, without emphasis. His role now was less to convince than to clarify edges already softening. The room didn't resist him anymore; it absorbed him. And absorption, he knew, was the precursor to permanence.

After the meeting, he stepped outside into the evening light. The air held a mildness that seemed to stretch the day by an extra hour, the last warmth of summer lingering in the breeze. Students moved across the quad in loose clusters, carrying backpacks, iced coffees, laughter.

He walked slowly toward the river path — not because he felt tired, but because the moment deserved the cadence of contemplation. He watched the water move beneath the footbridge, its surface calm, its current steady.

The work had entered a new stage:

neither struggle nor triumph,

but continuity.

The kind of continuity that breathes beyond a single life, beyond a single career, beyond a single scientific argument.

He rested both hands on the railing, letting the breeze move across his face, and understood something with full clarity:

He was no longer carrying the correction.

The correction was carrying itself.

There were early autumn evenings when the air carried that faint, unmistakable shift — the moment when warmth still lingered, but the light itself had begun to change. He felt it first in the angle of the sun, then in the way the shadows lengthened across the campus lawns, as though the world were preparing itself for a slower rhythm. These evenings always brought him a particular kind of clarity, the same clarity he felt in laboratories late at night or in conference rooms after everyone had left.

It wasn't nostalgia.

It wasn't melancholy.

It was recognition — the sense that something long in motion had reached another quiet waypoint.

On one such evening, he attended a modest roundtable discussion hosted by a regional public health collective. It was not a high-profile event; there were no keynote speakers, no elaborate graphics, no ceremonial introductions. Just a dozen professionals seated around a table with pitchers of water and loose stacks of papers. He liked gatherings like these — stripped of theatrics, stripped of hierarchy, stripped of the impulse to posture.

He took his seat and listened.

The conversation was already underway, a gentle debate about how best to revise community guidance for expectant mothers. One of the public health coordinators — a woman he had never met — leaned forward and said something without drama, without hesitation, without the slightest trace of inherited fear.

"I think we should retire the old language," she said. "It's misleading. And frankly, it's outdated. We know better now."

No one challenged her.

No one defended the old narrative.

No one asked for data to justify the transition.

The room simply agreed, the way a room agrees when the weather changes.

He didn't speak. He didn't need to. Someone else had carried the truth into the room before he arrived, and that was the most meaningful shift of all — the shift from his voice to theirs.

Later, as the group packed up its papers and exchanged the polite goodbyes of professionals accustomed to these small but significant gatherings, he stepped outside and felt the early autumn breeze move across the back of his neck. It was cooler now, enough to require a jacket, enough to suggest that the season was folding into the next.

He crossed the quiet parking lot toward his car, but something made him stop — not a sound, not a thought, but a sensation. A kind of interior stillness. He turned back toward the building and saw, through the glass doors, the faint reflection of the room he had just left. The chairs stacked neatly, the overhead lights dimming, the pitchers of water half-full.

It struck him then how profound the moment truly was.

Not the meeting itself.

Not the decision they made.

But the tone of it.

People were no longer waiting for permission to let go of the old warnings. They were no longer intimidated by the inertia of institutional history. They were no longer treating clarity as a disruption.

They were treating it as normal.

Normalcy — that was the true victory.

Not applause, not recognition, not policy endorsements.

Normalcy meant permanence.

Normalcy meant the correction had collapsed into the very structure of thought.

He stood there for a long moment, hands in his pockets, letting that recognition settle across him like a soft, cooling wind.

Then he noticed something else — something small but unmistakable.

A group of young residents walking out of the building, textbooks tucked under their arms, chatting lightly as they crossed the parking lot. He heard only a fragment of their conversation as they passed:

"...the protective factors matter more than the old warnings. It's a balance..."

That was enough.

Ordinary voices, unforced, carrying the truth forward without needing to reference his work, his name, or the long years it took to reach this point.

He started his car but didn't pull out right away. Instead, he watched the students walk toward the dimming horizon, their silhouettes framed by the last amber traces of daylight.

These were the inheritors.

Not of his career, but of the truth itself.

The truth he had protected long before anyone else would touch it.

The correction had crossed the boundary between knowledge and culture.

It now lived in everyday language, everyday practice, everyday decisions.

It lived in people who didn't know the history, didn't know the resistance, didn't know the decades of patience and restraint that had shaped it.

And that was exactly as it should be.

He shifted the car into gear, the headlights illuminating the quiet stretch of road ahead.

For the first time in a long time, he felt not the burden of stewardship —

but the calm of succession.

There were mid-autumn nights when he would leave the building later than planned, stepping into a world that had already surrendered to darkness. The campus, usually lively in the daylight hours, felt almost reverent at this time — the walkways empty, the lamps casting long, deliberate shadows, the air holding that cool, slightly metallic scent that appears only when the season begins its descent.

He liked the campus best at night.

The silence clarified things.

On one such evening, after a long discussion with a graduate student working on a thesis about nutrient interactions, he stepped out into the cool air and began walking toward the river path. His mind was still stirred by the conversation — not by anything the student had struggled with, but by what she had articulated effortlessly.

She had spoken about the selenium–mercury relationship with the ease of someone describing the structure of a familiar landscape. Not an argument. Not a discovery. A landscape.

He hadn't prompted it.

He hadn't guided her to it.

She simply understood it — as if the correction had always been there waiting for her.

He felt something inside him loosen.

It was a peculiar sensation, equal parts pride and distance — the realization that the truth had detached from him and migrated into the world with its own momentum. It no longer required his advocacy to survive. It no longer needed his voice to remain intact.

It had become self-protecting.

As he reached the river, he leaned on the cold railing of the footbridge and watched the reflections of campus lights shimmer on the dark surface. The water beneath moved quietly, carrying leaves in slow, irregular spirals. He had always liked how the river behaved at night — not loud, not dramatic, just steady.

He found himself thinking about the early years, when the resistance was subtle but constant — the raised eyebrows, the cautious tones, the polite skepticism that signaled people were willing to listen but not yet ready to understand. He remembered standing in rooms where every sentence felt like a small negotiation with the status quo. He remembered the interviews where he had to speak carefully, aware that the slightest misstep would be used to reinforce the old fears. He remembered the conferences where he sensed people agreeing privately but unwilling to contradict institutional directives in public.

And now — now the correction was slipping quietly into the structure of the world, leaving no trace of the struggle that had delivered it.

He continued walking along the path, moving slowly, not out of fatigue but out of a desire to remain inside this moment of quiet equilibrium. The leaves overhead rustled softly, some detaching, drifting down in broad arcs. A few landed gently on the river's surface, caught immediately by the current.

He thought of all the expectant mothers who had once avoided fish out of fear, all the children whose development had been shaped by old guidance that had equated complexity with danger. And then he thought of how many future children would never know those distortions — children who would benefit from a world offering proportion instead of panic, clarity instead of folklore.

This was the real meaning of the work:

Not the publications.

Not the lectures.

Not the decades of patience.

But the lives downstream — lives shaped by decisions informed not by fear, but by truth.

As he approached the end of the path, he saw a familiar figure standing near one of the benches — a colleague from another department, someone known more for environmental research than for nutritional science. They exchanged a quiet greeting, then the colleague said, without preamble:

“I’ve been reading some of the new advisories. They’re finally aligning with the balance you’ve been talking about all these years.”

There was no admiration in his tone.

No awe.

No surprise.

Just recognition.

The simplest and most honest form of acknowledgment.

“That’s good,” he replied. “It needed to happen.”

His colleague nodded in agreement, then added, "It changes how we talk about responsibility."

He didn't need to ask what he meant.

Responsibility was the quiet undercurrent of all public health guidance — the weight of shaping decisions for people who trusted institutions to speak clearly.

"Clarity is a form of responsibility," he said. "When we know better, we're obligated to say better."

The colleague accepted this with a thoughtful nod, then excused himself and walked back up the hill toward the campus buildings. He watched him go, the figure receding into the soft glow of the lamplights.

Standing there alone, he felt the subtle, undeniable truth settle inside him:

The world had begun to speak differently.

Not because he insisted.

Not because he repeated himself.

But because the truth had waited long enough for people to finally hear it.

He turned back toward the path, the autumn air cooling against his face, and walked slowly toward home.

The night around him was quiet.

The correction was steady.

The next movement was waiting.

There were mid-autumn afternoons when the light carried a kind of softened brilliance — angled, tempered, almost reflective — the sort of light that revealed details one might overlook in the height of summer. On days like this, he often found himself drawn to the far edge of campus where the older research buildings stood, their brickwork weathered by decades of prairie wind. These buildings, slightly removed from the main academic flow, always felt like places where thinking happened without performance.

He walked there now, hands in his pockets, letting the quiet settle over him.

Inside one of these older buildings, a small group of graduate students had gathered for an informal journal club. He wasn't scheduled to attend, but he had been invited with an open-ended "join us if you'd like," and today he felt inclined to accept. When he stepped into the room, they welcomed him with easy warmth — not the deferential caution he had once grown accustomed to, but the uncomplicated respect given to someone whose work had already woven itself into the underlying fabric of their understanding.

He sat near the back, listening.

The discussion that unfolded was sharper than he expected — not confrontational, but precise. They weren't wrestling with dogma. They were wrestling with nuance. A far better problem. One student pointed to how certain regions still lagged behind in updating their nutritional guidance. Another noted that maternal health literature still carried traces of old assumptions tucked between paragraphs.

But the most striking contribution came from a student who had been quiet until now, someone who seemed to be observing the conversation from a distance and measuring her words carefully.

"At some point," she said, "the world mistook simplicity for safety. And then it mistook fear for simplicity."

The room fell silent for a moment — not in awe, but in recognition.

He felt that silence land inside him with the gentle weight of truth.

He watched the conversation continue, branching in unexpected directions, connecting biochemical pathways to public messaging, molecular realities to cultural narratives. The students didn't frame their analysis as revolutionary. They framed it as necessary. And that distinction mattered. Necessary truths endure long after revolutionary truths fade.

When the session ended, they packed up their notebooks and thanked him for attending with the matter-of-fact tone reserved for a colleague, not a symbol. He appreciated that. He never wanted to be the center of the room; he only wanted the truth to be.

As he left the building, stepping back into the crisp air, he noticed a pair of posters pinned to the bulletin board near the exit. One advertised a seminar on nutrient synergy in early development. Another promoted a community outreach program focused on evidence-based prenatal nutrition. Neither bore his name. Neither referenced his work directly.

Yet both were unmistakably shaped by the correction he had devoted his life to.

He stood there for a long moment, studying the posters. Then he reached out and lightly touched the edge of one — not out of sentiment, but out of the quiet recognition that a world he once had to persuade now organized itself around a truth it had finally begun to trust.

He stepped outside, and the wind carried with it the scent of leaves just beginning to break down — that earthy, transitional smell that signaled the season's slow turn toward winter. Students moved in loose currents across the quad, their backpacks slung casually over one shoulder, their conversations drifting in the air like low murmurations.

He watched them for a moment, then continued down the path toward the river.

The light was thinning now, taking on a cooler tint. The water below moved with a kind of sober steadiness, its surface unbroken except for the occasional drifting leaf. He rested his hands on the railing and let his gaze soften.

There was no single moment when the world had changed.

No pivot point.

No dramatic revelation.

Instead, there had been thousands of small calibrations —

questions spoken in new tones,

sentences rewritten with new precision,

conversations held beneath elm trees,

committees revising language quietly,

students understanding the truth without being told it was once controversial.

It had not been a revolution.

It had been an accumulation.

And accumulations, he knew, were stronger.

He took a slow breath, letting the evening air settle into his lungs, and understood something with serene certainty: the work had reached a stage where each new movement was no longer an act of persuasion, but an act of refinement. The world wasn't just hearing the truth now — it was internalizing it.

He pushed gently off the railing and began the walk back toward campus, the leaves rustling at his feet, the sky deepening into early twilight.

The story was still unfolding.

But the foundation had become unshakeable.

There were early evenings in late autumn when the buildings on campus seemed to glow from within — not brightly, but with a kind of interior steadiness, like lanterns holding their own modest center of warmth against the lengthening night. He often found himself lingering outside these buildings before going in, listening to the faint hum of HVAC systems and the soft echo of distant footsteps moving through near-empty corridors. The world felt slower at this hour, as though it were holding still long enough for deeper truths to register.

He stepped inside one of the academic wings and made his way toward a seminar room where a small interdisciplinary panel was being held. It wasn't a high-profile gathering — no polished signage, no formal introductions — just a circle of chairs, a carafe of coffee cooling on a side table, and a dozen people who cared enough about clarity to show up after hours.

He slipped into a seat near the back and listened.

The panel topic was not nutrition, at least not directly. It was about the responsibility of expertise — how fields should respond when long-held public guidance turns out to be incomplete. A sociologist spoke first, describing the difficulty institutions have with correction. A communication specialist followed, explaining how narratives become self-protecting. And then a public health professor — someone he had known casually for years — leaned forward and said something that made the room pause.

"There's an example in our own community," she said. "A long-standing cautionary message about diet during pregnancy — repeated everywhere, taught everywhere — that turned out to be missing half the truth. The problem wasn't malice. It was momentum."

He felt that word settle in the room.

Momentum.

A force nobody sees until it resists change.

She continued:

"We spent years telling mothers what not to eat instead of teaching them what the body actually needs. And we did it because fear is easier to communicate than proportion."

No one disagreed.

No one even shifted uncomfortably.

It was simply acknowledged, absorbed, accepted.

For a moment he wondered whether anyone would look toward him, or gesture to him, or reference him by implication. But no one did. And that — surprisingly, beautifully — felt exactly right.

The correction had become larger than him.

It did not require his presence to exist.

It did not require his name to be credible.

Someone else in the room added quietly, "Science doesn't fail when it changes. It fails when it refuses to."

The conversation expanded from there — into ethics, communication, the subtle difference between authority and clarity. He said little. He didn't need to. The field was speaking in a voice that no longer needed his guidance.

When the session ended, people gathered their coats and papers, exchanging small comments as they drifted toward the exit. He lingered for a moment, watching the slow dispersal of colleagues into the hallway, each carrying some piece of renewed perspective.

As he stepped into the crisp night air, he felt an odd mixture of distance and belonging — the sensation of someone who had spent years shaping a landscape only to find, at last, that the landscape now shaped itself.

He walked across the quiet quad toward the northern footpath, where the trees formed a canopy of branches now mostly bare. The leaves that remained clung not out of defiance, but out of timing — nature's own slow relinquishment. He watched one leaf detach and drift downward, its motion slow, deliberate, almost ceremonial.

He found himself thinking about the earliest days of his work — the forgotten conference rooms, the handwritten notes, the quiet frustrations, the hesitant questions. It all felt distant now, almost archival, as though it belonged not to his memory but to some earlier version of the world.

And yet the path from then to now was exquisitely clear.

Not linear.

Not smooth.

But clear.

He reached the river overlook and paused, resting both hands on the railing. The water below moved with a dark, reflective calm, rippling under the faint glow of campus lights. He watched the surface shift — fractured reflections, subtle distortions, small currents rearranging patterns.

It reminded him of the way understanding changed:

not all at once, but in layers.

Not with declarations, but with adjustments.

Not through argument, but through quiet recognition.

He exhaled slowly, the warm breath drifting visibly into the cool air.

The work was no longer a weight he carried.

It was a truth the world was finally learning to hold.

He stayed there for a long moment, letting the silence gather around him, then turned toward the path that led back through campus — walking with a calm certainty that the next movement would unfold exactly when and how it needed to.

There were evenings when the horizon dimmed into a muted violet, the kind of color that appears only in the last hour before night fully settles. He always noticed that shade — not because it was beautiful (though it was), but because it carried the same quality that defined the later stages of his work: a softness that arrived only after years of intensity. A quiet earned, not given.

He walked along the north edge of campus during one such evening, the grass cool beneath his shoes, the lamplight stretching out in narrow gold bands across the pavement. Students passed him in clusters, laughing, talking, unaware that the ground they walked on — intellectually, structurally — had shifted beneath them in ways they would never need to trace.

As he approached the older wing of the science complex, he saw a doorway half-open, light spilling into the hallway in a narrow, diagonal beam. Voices drifted out — not loud, not formal, just the sound of animated discussion. He paused, listening not to the words themselves but to the cadence: earnest, exploratory, unburdened.

He stepped inside quietly.

A small group of faculty members were gathered around a whiteboard, discussing updates to their introductory curriculum for undergraduate health science students. He recognized some of them; others were new faces, younger, perhaps recently hired. They were rewriting modules on maternal nutrition, refining outdated sections, debating how much biochemical detail early students could reasonably absorb.

He didn't speak. He simply listened.

One of the younger faculty members was outlining a draft for a new lecture, circling terms on the board with a marker: nutrient synergy, fetal protection, molecular context. The phrasing struck him — not because it was revolutionary, but because it was unselfconscious. These were not people nervous about challenging a myth. These were people who had grown up inside a world already shedding it.

At one point, a professor he had known for years said, "We need to make this material evidence-forward. Students should understand how the protective factors actually work, not just hear simplified warnings based on outdated models."

Another added, "Avoidance isn't a teaching strategy. Context is."

No one argued.

No one hesitated.

No one invoked the old narratives.

He felt a shift inside him, subtle but unmistakable — a recognition that the correction was now embedded at the architectural level. Not in special seminars. Not in advanced research groups. But in the entryway of education, the very place where future clinicians first formed their instincts.

He watched the discussion unfold for a few minutes more before stepping back into the hallway. The door closed behind him with a soft click, leaving him alone in the wide, quiet corridor. He began walking slowly, feeling the cool floor underfoot, the building's familiar hum vibrating faintly through the walls.

Halfway down the hall, he stopped at a display case filled with artifacts from decades past — old lab instruments, weathered notebooks, photographs of early faculty members. He had passed this case thousands of times, rarely giving it more than a glance. But tonight, something made him pause.

He leaned in, studying an old black-and-white photograph of a nutrition lecture from the 1970s. Rows of students sat in rigid posture, taking notes while a professor diagrammed a biochemical pathway on a chalkboard. The students looked earnest, curious — but the framework they were inheriting had not yet understood the molecular interaction he would one day devote his life to.

He stared at the photograph and felt a strange sense of temporal layering — the past uncorrected, the present correcting, the future already aligned.

He lifted his gaze and saw his own faint reflection in the glass — not as a figure in the center of the frame, but as a quiet presence somewhere at the periphery. And that, he realized, was exactly where he belonged now.

The center had shifted.

The narrative had relocated.

The truth had migrated into places that no longer required him to stand guard over it.

He walked out of the building and into the evening air, the sky now deepening toward blue-black. Leaves rustled overhead, some breaking free and drifting down with the slow, spiraling grace that only autumn can produce.

He stood there for a moment, letting the night settle around him.

There was no milestone to celebrate.

No announcement to mark.

No single moment to point to and say: Here. This is where everything changed.

Because it hadn't changed in one place.

It had changed everywhere, quietly, cumulatively, faithfully.

He felt the calm certainty of someone who had spent a lifetime tending a flame that no longer needed tending.

The correction was alive.

The world had matured enough to hold it.

And the next movement — whatever it would be — would not require force.

It would require only presence.

He turned toward the footpath that led home, walking slowly beneath the lamplight, each step steady, deliberate, assured.

There were certain winter evenings when the cold descended not as an announcement but as a quiet claiming — a gradual tightening of the air that made every breath feel a little sharper, every sound a little clearer, every movement a little more precise. On nights like this, he often found himself returning to the long glass corridor that connected two of the science buildings. It was a place he had walked through hundreds of times, but in winter it became something else entirely.

The corridor acted like a lens.

Inside, the air was warm, the lights low, the glass panels stretching out on both sides like parallel sheets of darkened water. Outside, snow drifted across the empty campus in slow, diagonal lines, illuminated by the lamplight with the soft luminance of falling ash.

He paused halfway down the corridor, his reflection faint and layered in the glass. In the dimness, he could see trees bending in the wind, their branches skeletal and unadorned — honest, unembellished forms. Winter stripped things down to their essence. He liked that about it. Clarity always appeared when ornament fell away.

Behind him, two graduate instructors walked past, speaking in low voices about the revisions to next semester's curriculum.

"...the protective mechanisms should be introduced earlier," one said. "If students learn the balance from the start, the old assumptions won't have room to take hold."

The other nodded. "We should treat clarity as foundational, not corrective."

He stood still, listening to the way their words blended with the soft hum of the corridor's heating system. Once, long ago, he would have felt compelled to intervene, to shape the conversation, to press the urgency of what they were now discussing as casually as weather. Now he found comfort in the fact that he was invisible to the conversation — unnecessary, in the best possible way.

He continued walking until he reached the west exit, where a set of glass doors faced the open quad. The wind outside moved in long, sweeping gusts. Snow lifted from the ground in low spirals, dancing across the pavement before settling again. The lampposts flickered slightly, their light haloed in the frost.

He stepped out into the cold.

The air hit him with that pure, crystalline chill known only to northern plains winters — the kind that clarified the senses without punishing them. His breath rose in small plumes as he crossed the quad, the snow crunching sharply beneath his boots.

The campus was nearly empty.

Winter did that — it made silence into a kind of architecture.

As he approached the edge of the river path, he noticed a single light glowing in one of the small community education buildings near the water. Someone was still working inside, long after most people had gone home. He recognized the silhouette of a young outreach coordinator — someone tasked with updating the county's maternal nutrition materials for the coming year.

He hesitated for a moment, then walked toward the building.

Inside, she was seated at a long table, surrounded by drafts, diagrams, and sticky notes. When she looked up and saw him, she smiled with the easy, unguarded familiarity of someone who considered him less an icon and more a colleague.

"I'm trying to simplify the section on micronutrient balance," she said, gesturing to the papers spread before her. "We want it to be accessible but accurate. The old materials relied too much on avoidance language. We're changing that."

He leaned over the table, scanning the draft. He noticed something remarkable — not in the wording itself, but in the rhythm of the sentences. They carried proportion. They carried confidence. They carried none of the timidity that had once shadowed every attempt to shift public messaging.

"You've framed it well," he said. "You're giving people the truth in a way they can actually absorb."

She nodded. "People are ready to understand it."

He wasn't sure if that statement was meant as reassurance or observation, but it didn't matter. It was true either way.

He stood there for a long moment, the warmth of the room settling into his winter-chilled bones, the hum of a small desk lamp casting a soft glow across the drafts. Then he stepped back, offering a small nod of encouragement before heading toward the door.

"Thank you for this," she said quietly as he reached for the handle.

He paused. "You're the one doing the work now."

Outside, the wind carried flakes of snow sideways, brushing against his face as he began the walk back toward campus. The night had grown colder, the sky deepening into a muted slate. He felt the snow settling onto his coat, melting slowly with each step.

It occurred to him then — gently, without weight — that the world no longer required him to fight for the truth he had spent his life defending. It required only that he continue to witness its unfolding.

He walked on, the river murmuring faintly under its thin crust of early ice, the winter air sharpening the edges of the evening into crystalline precision.

The correction had survived the season.

And the season had finally begun to speak its language.

There were late-winter mornings when the sun rose not as a triumphant blaze but as a pale, deliberate disc — a light that arrived with restraint, as though it were measuring the world before engaging it. On mornings like this, he often found himself awake earlier than expected, moving through the quiet house with a kind of contemplative alertness. The kettle heating, the soft creak of floorboards, the slow unfolding of the day — everything felt calibrated, precise.

He would pour his coffee, put on his coat, and walk to campus before most offices had unlocked their doors.

The air held a cold so fine it felt almost clean.

A clarity without cruelty.

He crossed the nearly empty quad, the snow crusted over from several freeze-thaw cycles, shimmering like glass in the early light. His footsteps left shallow impressions that quickly filled with fresh powder drifting sideways on the wind. He entered the sciences building through a side door he had used for years — a habit formed less from necessity than from familiarity.

Inside, the building was still warming itself awake.

As he made his way down the hall, he noticed a light coming from one of the smaller conference rooms. Curious, he glanced through the narrow window in the door. A group of second-year medical students were gathered around a table, their laptops open, their coffee cups half-empty, their expression the universal look of young professionals preparing for an exam that mattered deeply.

They were studying prenatal care.

He stepped inside quietly, offering a polite nod as the students straightened in their seats. Their instructor — a younger clinician whose work he respected — greeted him warmly and gestured for him to join them if he wished.

He took a seat at the edge of the room, listening.

The students were reviewing case studies, some based on real scenarios, others theoretical. One case involved a pregnant patient uncertain about seafood consumption. The students discussed it with a fluency that would have been nearly unimaginable years ago.

One said, “We need to understand the nutrient profile, not just the perceived risk.”

Another added, “If selenium is adequate, the protective mechanisms are stable. The concern isn’t about the presence of mercury — it’s about the absence of balance.”

A third student — soft-spoken, thoughtful — summarized the case with quiet confidence:

"We should emphasize nourishment instead of avoidance. Fear-based guidance causes more harm than biochemical reality."

The instructor nodded. "Exactly. Our responsibility is to give mothers clarity, not caution without context."

He watched them speak, their discussions unburdened by hesitation, their reasoning aligned with truths he once had to defend point by point. There was no performance here, no need for rhetorical finesse. These students were not merely repeating information — they were integrating it, reasoning with it, carrying it forward.

He felt something in his chest shift — not pride, not relief, but a deeper sense of continuity.

The kind that arrives only when you see the future behaving as though your work had always been part of its architecture.

At the end of the session, as the students gathered their belongings and filed out into the hallway, one lingered for a moment. She approached him with a mixture of curiosity and respect.

"I just wanted to say," she began, "I used to hear so much conflicting information. But when I learned the actual chemistry behind it — the real balance — it suddenly made sense. It felt... fair. Like the body wasn't the enemy."

He regarded her for a moment, recognizing the earnestness in her expression — the earnestness of someone who had crossed the threshold from confusion to clarity.

"The body rarely is," he said. "It's usually the narratives that are."

She smiled softly, thanked him, and hurried out to join her classmates.

He stayed in the room a moment longer, alone now in the warm quiet. The window looked out over the river, where thin sheets of ice were beginning to fragment, drifting apart in slow, deliberate movements. Winter was loosening its grip. The season of correction — both literal and metaphorical — was giving way to something more fluid.

He stepped back into the hallway, the building now awakened with footsteps and voices, and walked toward his office with a calm he had rarely felt in earlier years. For the first time, he sensed the world was not merely catching up — it was preparing to move ahead.

The work had entered a phase beyond stewardship.

It had entered a phase of inheritance.

He opened his office door, set down his coffee, and breathed in the stillness before the day fully began.

There were early spring afternoons when the wind carried the faintest promise of warmth, though the snow still clung stubbornly to the north-facing edges of buildings and the bare soil beneath the trees lay dark and damp. These in-between days were never loud in their arrival. They announced themselves through subtleties — the softened light, the smell of thawing earth, the quiet restlessness of students who sensed a change before they could name it.

He walked across campus during one such afternoon, the sun hanging low but bright, the sidewalks crowded with melting ice that crackled softly underfoot. The world felt like it was rewriting itself, and he could not help noticing the parallel.

Inside the biomedical wing, a small symposium was underway. Not a grand event — no banners, no catered lunch — but a working session of researchers sharing data from the field. He slipped into the lecture hall, taking a seat in the back row, watching the glow of slides move across the screen at the front.

A young researcher was presenting preliminary findings from a study in a rural clinic network. The graphs were simple — uptake patterns, dietary surveys, developmental markers — but the shapes of the lines spoke volumes. The audience leaned in, not because the conclusions were dramatic, but because they were coherent.

The researcher, adjusting his glasses, said calmly:

"We expected resistance to updated nutritional guidance, but instead we found the opposite. When the information is presented with clarity — not alarm, not ambiguity — mothers are receptive. The limiting factor isn't fear. It's accuracy."

He felt a stillness settle through the room.

Another slide appeared — a scatter plot showing maternal nutrient profiles over time. The clustering was clear. The protective balance held. The developmental outcomes were consistent.

A clinician raised her hand.

“So you’re saying,” she asked, “that when we correct the narrative, people adjust faster than we predicted?”

The researcher nodded. “Once they understand the mechanism, yes. The correction becomes intuitive.”

That word — intuitive — struck him.

For years, intuition had been the obstacle.

Now it had become the ally.

When the session concluded, he stepped into the hallway, where a few attendees had gathered in small groups, murmuring about implications for public health messaging. Their tone wasn’t breathless, nor defensive, nor cautious. It was matter-of-fact.

He walked slowly toward the exit, passing the framed photographs of faculty members from decades past. As he reached the atrium, he saw a poster on the wall — an advertisement for an upcoming seminar titled “Nutrient Equilibrium in Early Brain Development.”

Below the title was a subheading:

A Modern Framework for Maternal Seafood Consumption.

No references to fear.

No hedging language.

No inherited caution.

Just a straightforward acknowledgment that the framework had shifted.

He paused for a moment, reading the description. The wording was elegant in its simplicity — an invitation rather than a warning. A doorway rather than a barrier.

Outside, the snowmelt created thin streams that trickled along the edges of the sidewalk, carrying bits of debris — leaves, grit, fragments of winter — toward the storm drains. He found himself stopping near one of these small rivulets, watching the water thread its way through the uneven pavement toward a drain partially obscured by slush.

It reminded him of the way truth moved:

not always quickly,

not always cleanly,

but inevitably, following the path gravity carved for it.

He crossed the street toward the older research buildings, where the river trail curved behind the campus. The water was still partly iced over, but cracks had begun to appear, long fissures forming delicate lace-like patterns. Underneath, the current whispered against the underside of the thawing ice.

He stood there, listening.

Winter was loosening its hold in slow, articulate ways — the same way institutions loosened their grip on outdated narratives, the same way minds surrendered old fears once they saw the proportions clearly.

He realized, standing there by the river, that the shift he had once imagined would require a lifetime might instead materialize through the next generation. Not through force, but through recognition. Not through debate, but through proportion.

Far behind him, the hallways of the university hummed with new language.

Ahead of him, the river carried winter away in small dissolving sheets.

The world was learning how to speak the correction without needing to rehearse it.

He felt neither release nor triumph — only a kind of quiet verification, like hearing an echo return in the exact tone in which it was sent.

Spring was arriving.

And with it, a world finally prepared to move forward without hesitation.

There were late-spring mornings when the world felt impossibly clean, as though the previous night's rain had rinsed the air of every remnant of winter. The sky carried that pale, translucent blue that appears only in the earliest hours of the season, before the heat has begun its slow ascent. He always noticed those mornings — not because they were dramatic, but because they marked a kind of reset. A quiet renewal that required no announcement.

He crossed the parking lot toward the research wing, the asphalt still darkened by rain, small puddles reflecting slices of sky. Birds were louder now; students walked with lighter steps; the trees, newly leafed, murmured in the wind with the soft confidence of things emerging from a long sleep.

Inside the building, the hallways were alive with a different kind of energy — not the hurried tension of midterm season, but the anticipatory rhythm of upcoming conferences, grant proposals, and summer research rotations. Posters lined the walls, showcasing undergraduate projects and graduate theses. Some were expected; others were new.

He stopped in front of one he hadn't seen before.

It was a simple layout — no embellishment, no overreaching claims. The title read:

"Maternal Seafood Consumption: Evaluating Protective Nutrient Ratios in Rural Communities."

Below it, student authors were listed alongside their faculty advisor. He skimmed the abstract — concise, balanced, and unmistakably grounded in the corrected framework. What struck him most was the tone. There was no defensiveness, no hint of caution around the subject. The students spoke as though they were operating inside a truth already established.

And they were.

He continued down the hall toward a seminar room where a team meeting was scheduled. This wasn't his team, but he had been invited to sit in — a courtesy extended to someone whose perspective still carried weight, even if it no longer shaped the center of gravity. He appreciated these invitations for what they represented: not reverence, but integration.

When he entered, a small group of postdoctoral researchers were already gathered around the table, laptops open, documents spread out in front of them. They were preparing a presentation for an interdisciplinary symposium — one that would bring together nutritionists, environmental scientists, pediatricians, and policy analysts.

He listened as they rehearsed.

One postdoc was explaining how early developmental brain protection depended not on the presence or absence of any single element, but on the competing demands of biochemical priorities. She spoke clearly, without ornament, in the calm voice of someone who understood the proportion instinctively.

Another researcher added, “The misconception persisted because the guidance focused on what we feared instead of what we needed. We want the symposium to illustrate that correction isn’t reversal — it’s refinement.”

He felt the room deepen in its focus.

They were not repeating his language.

They were creating their own.

The meeting continued, each voice contributing a piece of a larger mosaic. And as he listened, he sensed something subtle but unmistakable: the correction had reached a point of cultural fluency. Not universal, not complete — but fluent.

When the rehearsal ended, one of the researchers turned to him.

“Would you change anything?” she asked. Not deferentially — collaboratively.

He considered the question, then shook his head slightly.

“No. You’re asking the right questions now. That’s what matters.”

They nodded, satisfied, and returned to refining their slides.

He stepped out of the room and into the sunlight streaming through tall windows in the atrium. The light had shifted — warmer now, fuller, more assured. Students crossed the quad outside, talking, laughing, navigating the end of the semester with that mixture of exhaustion and exhilaration familiar to campuses everywhere.

He walked through the glass doors and descended the wide concrete steps that led back toward the river path. The breeze carried the smell of damp soil and budding grass. Along the river, the last shards of ice had finally dissolved, leaving the water dark, smooth, and unobstructed — a continuous surface reflecting an unbroken sky.

He stopped at the railing and rested his hands there, watching the current move. It was faster now, energized by the melt upstream. Clearer, too.

He realized that clarity always arrived downstream — after the turbulence, after the uncertainty, after the long winter of resistance. What mattered was not the swiftness but the inevitability.

And in that moment, he understood the work in its truest form:

It was not a fight.

Not an argument.

Not a crusade.

It was a long calibration — molecular, institutional, generational — that had finally begun to hold its shape.

He listened to the river, its steady movement mirroring the quiet certainty that now lived inside him.

Spring had taken hold.

And the world, at last, was fluent in its own proportions.

There were early summer evenings when the day refused to end — lingering, stretching, holding itself open as though the light were reluctant to leave. On evenings like this, campus felt suspended in a kind of gentle equilibrium. Students were gone, the academic year concluded, and yet the place still carried a pulse — not loud, not busy, but alive in the way landscapes remain alive after the people have stepped aside.

He walked along the central quad, the grass thick and brilliantly green, the air warm enough that he didn't need a jacket but cool enough that the heat of July still felt distant. The sky had that long, unbroken gradient from pale gold near the horizon to a deeper blue overhead. He always liked this time of year — the intermission between demands.

Inside the research building, the corridors were mostly dark except for a few scattered lights from offices where summer projects had quietly resumed. He passed by one open door and heard the soft clatter of someone typing, the shifting of papers, the small movements of concentration. It reminded him of his own early years — work continuing through the edges of seasons, driven not by deadlines but by the steady pull of curiosity.

He kept walking.

Near the end of the hall, he saw something unexpected: a group of high school students on a summer STEM program, clustered around a table with an instructor explaining basic nutrient interactions. Their voices were excited in that particular way only young minds can be — unfiltered, earnest, unselfconscious.

He paused near the doorway.

The instructor — someone he didn't recognize — was sketching a simple diagram on a whiteboard: a protective nutrient, a competing element, a balance that determined outcome. It wasn't sophisticated, but it was accurate. More importantly, it was intuitive in the way it was being presented.

A student raised her hand.

"So... it's not that one thing is bad?"

"Correct," the instructor said. "It's about what the body prioritizes. If the protective factor is present, development stays on course."

Another student jumped in.

"Then why did they used to say not to eat fish?"

The instructor paused — not awkwardly, but thoughtfully.

"Sometimes guidance starts with fear instead of proportion," she said. "And it takes time for the world to correct its footing."

He could've smiled, but he didn't. Instead, he simply watched the students absorbing the idea — not as a controversy, but as clarity. They were too young to remember the old warnings, too young to inherit the anxieties that had shaped earlier generations. They were receiving the truth without ever having carried the myth.

He left them to their learning and stepped back into the hallway, walking toward the exit.

Outside, the air felt warmer now, carrying the sweet scent of blooming clover and the faint hum of insects rising with the dusk. He followed the path toward the river, where the sun was lowering itself into a long shimmer across the surface of the water. The current had slowed from the spring rush — calm now, deliberate, its surface moving with a quiet confidence that matched the season.

He approached the railing and leaned forward slightly, letting the soft orange light reflect on his hands.

The river always helped him think.

Not about the past — he no longer felt the old need to revisit the early battles — but about the shape of things now. How different the world looked when the truth no longer needed a shield. How quietly, how elegantly, the next generation took hold of what had been painstakingly protected.

He listened to the lapping water below, the faint voices of a few students on bicycles passing behind him, the low hum of distant traffic blending into the evening. Everything felt balanced — not in some grand philosophical sense, but in a way that suggested continuity had become effortless.

He thought of the decades — the early frustrations, the loneliness of being out of step with an entrenched narrative, the careful explanations given to rooms not yet ready to hear them. And then the slow thaw — one mind at a time, one revised document at a time, one recalibrated instinct at a time.

And now, here he was, standing in a world where the correction no longer needed his presence to survive.

A world fluent in its own equilibrium.

He stepped back from the railing and began walking up the hill toward the heart of campus, the last of the sunlight catching the tops of the buildings in a soft, amber glow. His pace was unhurried. There was no urgency anymore. The work had transcended urgency. It existed now in a stable orbit.

As he reached the top of the hill, the lights across campus flickered on in unison. The world seemed to exhale.

Summer had taken hold.

And with it came a quiet truth:

the next movement would not be shaped by resistance, but by understanding.

There were midsummer nights when the air held a softness so complete it felt almost like a presence — warm, steady, unbroken. On nights like this, the campus transformed into something quieter, almost contemplative. The buildings that bustled during the academic year now stood as tall silhouettes against a pale, lingering twilight. The walkways were empty except for the occasional faculty member heading home late or a lone student finishing a summer lab rotation.

He liked to walk during these hours, when the world had unspooled its noise and the light hovered in that narrow place between day and dark.

He found himself crossing the lawn behind the environmental sciences building, where a stand of old trees created a small clearing. The grass was cool beneath his shoes, the breeze warm against his face. Fireflies flickered near the edge of the clearing, tiny lanterns drifting in and out of visibility — faint, ephemeral, persistent.

He followed the path toward the river, hearing in the distance the soft hum of an outdoor generator powering a temporary research tent. Summer projects tended to spill out of buildings — field testing equipment, portable labs, graduate students mapping soil or water sampling sites. The university in summer felt less like an institution and more like a living workshop.

As he neared the riverbank, he saw a group of graduate fellows gathered around a folding table, their laptops open, a few lanterns casting gentle halos of light around them. They were discussing data from a community outreach project — maternal dietary patterns collected across several counties, cross-referenced with developmental markers and environmental factors.

He stopped a few steps away, not wanting to interrupt, but they waved him over with the ease of people who saw him not as a distant figure but as part of their landscape.

"We're analyzing trend shifts over the last decade," one of the fellows said, turning a laptop toward him. "It's fascinating. The old avoidance patterns have decreased significantly. People are choosing based on benefit now, not fear."

Another added, "What surprises me most is how quickly the shift happened once the messaging changed. People weren't resistant — they were waiting."

Waiting.

That word lingered in the warm air.

He studied the data. The lines were clean, the clusters tight, the trend unmistakable. It wasn't flashy — good science never was — but it told a long, patient story. A story of recalibration. A story of proportion taking root. A story of cultural instinct correcting itself.

"People adapt faster than institutions do," he said quietly, almost to himself.

One of the fellows nodded. "Because people are allowed to be curious. Institutions think they have to be cautious."

They continued discussing the data, layering insights, refining interpretations, tracing implications. As he listened, he felt the familiar blend of distance and belonging — the recognition of a world moving forward without needing his hand on its shoulder.

After a while, the group began to pack up their equipment, laughing softly, making plans for tomorrow's session. He left them to their work and walked toward the water's edge.

The river at night was a darker version of its daytime self — slower, heavier, more reflective. The surface caught the moonlight in long, trembling ribbons. He stood on the bank, hands clasped loosely behind him, letting the warm breeze drift across his face.

Above him, the sky deepened into a vast, quiet expanse — no longer the bright canvas of day but a softer, more deliberate backdrop. The constellations were just beginning to appear, faint but certain.

He looked up and felt a rare, steady kind of recognition:

The truth had finally settled into the world the way seasons settle into each other — gradually, then fully.

Not through force.

Not through argument.

But through inevitability.

He listened to the nighttime insects humming in the grass, to the distant laughter of the graduate fellows walking back toward campus, to the river's quiet, ceaseless conversation with the shoreline.

Clarity had become a condition of the landscape.

He turned away from the river and began walking back up the hill, the warm night air moving gently around him. There was no rush. No pressure. The next movement would arrive not through urgency, but through continuation.

And as he reached the crest of the hill, he paused to take in the entire campus — dimly lit, softly humming, alive in its quiet way — and understood that this was what the long work had been moving toward all along:

A world in which the truth did not need a guardian.

Only witnesses.

There were late-summer dawns when the light rose without ceremony, sliding quietly over the horizon in a thin, silver band that touched the tops of buildings before it reached the ground. These mornings had a kind of suspended clarity — a pause before the day began in earnest, as though the world were letting its structure show through before covering itself again with movement and noise.

He found himself awake before sunrise on such a morning, drawn by habit rather than obligation. The house was still, the air faintly cool. He brewed his coffee in silence, listening to the soft hiss of the kettle, then stepped outside and began walking toward campus.

The streets were empty except for a lone maintenance truck moving slowly along the curb, its amber light rotating in steady rhythm. The surrounding houses — professors' homes, rental units for graduate students, small apartments tucked between trees — were dark except for the occasional lamp left on overnight.

He reached the university just as the first edge of sunlight touched the highest windows.

Everything felt newly made.

He crossed the quad, the grass still damp from the night, the leaves rustling faintly in the initial stirrings of the breeze. The buildings stood in that early light with a kind of architectural sincerity — their lines clean, their edges defined, their histories intact but unspoken.

He walked toward the biomedical annex, where a summer workshop was scheduled to begin later in the day. He was not leading it — they no longer needed him to — but he had been invited to stop by if he wished. He arrived early on purpose. He preferred to see rooms before they filled, preferred to sense the quiet intention a space held before the conversations began.

Inside, the seminar room was partially set up. A projector hummed softly to itself; a stack of handouts lay neatly arranged on a table; the windows were open just enough to let the morning breeze carry in the scent of dewy grass. He wandered toward the podium, not to inspect it, but to feel the atmosphere of a room prepared for clarity.

He noticed a slide already queued on the screen:

"Maternal Nutrition: Correcting the Vector of Misunderstanding."

He read the title twice.

Not because it surprised him — but because it didn't.

A researcher entered the room carrying a box of cables and adapters. She greeted him warmly, without the slightest trace of the old guardedness people once adopted around his work, and began arranging her materials.

"You're early," she said with a smile.

"I wanted to see the room before it woke up," he replied.

She nodded, understanding exactly what he meant. Then she said something that stayed with him long after the conversation ended:

"We've moved past reacting to the old guidance. Now we're building the new one."

He stood there, letting the meaning settle.

Building the new one.

That was the shift — the true shift.

Not dismantling the past.

Not defending the correction.

Not persuading reluctant minds.

But building onward.

He stayed for the first part of the workshop, seated quietly in the back. The instructors spoke with a calm, measured confidence, explaining the protective interplay of nutrients with the ease of people discussing established physics. The participants — a mix of clinicians, nutritionists, and community health workers — asked thoughtful questions, not about fear, but about implementation.

“How do we teach this?” one asked.

“How do we update our materials without overwhelming people?” another added.

He thought of the decades when the questions had been entirely different — questions rooted in caution, anxiety, inherited assumptions. Now the questions were forward-facing. Constructive. Practical.

The world was no longer asking whether the correction was real.

It was asking how to operationalize it.

When the workshop reached its midpoint, he stepped outside, wanting to walk while the day was still new. The sky had brightened fully now, the sun clearing the rooftops, warming the tops of the tallest trees first. The shadows were long but soft.

He followed the familiar path down to the river.

The summer water was calm — not sluggish, but settled. A few birds dotted the shoreline; the leaves on the overhanging branches shook lightly in the warm breeze. He leaned on the railing, watching the current take its time.

The river had changed over the seasons — frozen, thawed, rushed, slowed — yet always maintained its direction. He knew the work had followed the same pattern: long cycles of resistance, long cycles of recalibration, long cycles of quiet realignment.

And now, finally, a season of steady flow.

He stood there listening to the soft sounds of water against the bank. The breeze moved through the trees with an ease that belonged only to late August — neither the urgency of spring nor the heaviness of midsummer, but something in between. A balance.

He understood then, with calm certainty, that the work had entered the stage he once wondered if he would live to see: a stage where clarity no longer needed to fight for a place at the table.

It simply was the table.

He turned back toward campus, the morning now fully awake, the buildings catching the sun with a quiet, confident glow.

The next movement waited in the day ahead.

There were late-summer afternoons when the air felt warm enough to suggest the season was steady, only for a stray pocket of coolness to pass through — a reminder that transitions were never as clean as calendars pretended. He felt that same unevenness in the people he encountered. The young, with their straightforward acceptance. The older, with their layered memories of warnings recited so often they had become reflex.

He noticed it now as he crossed the quad.

Ahead of him, a retired faculty member — someone he had known for years — stood by the benches, engaged in conversation with a former colleague. Their voices carried just enough for him to catch fragments.

"...I still worry about exposure..."

"...we didn't have all this nuance back then..."

"...some things are better left cautious..."

He slowed his pace — not to eavesdrop, but to observe the familiar cadence of a generation whose instincts had been shaped by decades of messaging that had never made room for proportion. They weren't stubborn. They weren't ignorant. They were simply inhabiting the ghosts of earlier frameworks.

As he passed them, they nodded politely, with the warm but reserved familiarity of people who respected him yet remained tethered to their own certainty.

He kept walking.

The wind shifted, warm again, as though the cool pocket had been nothing more than a passing lapse. Ahead, a group of undergraduates sat on the grass beneath an elm tree, eating lunch, scrolling through their tablets, talking casually. One of them mentioned an assignment in a nutrition class.

"It makes sense," she said. "You look at the whole profile, not just one part. I don't get why they made such a big deal about it before."

He caught only that line as he walked by, but it was enough.

The divide between the two conversations — fifty feet apart, decades in worldview — could not have been clearer.

As he reached the sidewalk leading toward the sciences wing, he felt the air steady again. The weather was doing what the world was doing: fluctuating, correcting, drifting between temperatures old and new. The campus trees rustled above him in a pattern that almost resembled speech — sporadic, layered, half-formed phrases carried on the breeze.

Inside the building, the hallway lights flickered softly awake as motion sensors detected his presence. He walked past an open office door where two mid-career clinicians were discussing updates to state guidelines. Their tone was measured, professional, but each sentence carried a kind of cautious friction — the sound of people recalibrating without fully admitting they were recalibrating.

“Do you think patients will understand the shift?”

“They will if we frame it right.”

“I’m just not sure the board is ready.”

He paused, unseen, long enough to feel the atmosphere of the conversation: not resistance, not acceptance, but negotiation. A generation standing on a threshold with one foot in each world.

He moved on.

Down the hall, he entered the atrium, where sunlight streamed through the tall glass windows, illuminating dust motes suspended in the warm air like fragments of thought not yet anchored. A digital screen displayed an announcement for an upcoming symposium. Beneath it, a scrolling banner read:

"Emerging Paradigms in Maternal Nutrition: Balancing Risk and Reality."

And there it was again — that soft echo of the old framework, trying to hold on through the language of caution. "Balancing risk."

Not wrong.

Not right.

Just incomplete.

He stood there for a long moment, the sunlight warming his shoulders as he listened to the quiet debates occurring on opposite ends of the building, in opposite ends of the generational spectrum. One conversation moving with the ease of a world that had already crossed the threshold. The other still bracing itself on the old vocabulary.

He didn't judge either. He simply recognized the weather of it — the familiar fluctuations of transition.

A warm breeze, then a cool pocket.

A moment of clarity, then an instinctive retreat.

A world correcting itself, but unevenly.

He understood this rhythm.

He had lived inside it for decades.

And as he stepped back onto the walkway outside, he felt the warm air reclaim the afternoon as though the coolness had never existed. Students laughed in the distance. A faculty member walked briskly toward the library. A maintenance cart rumbled across the pavement.

The season held, but only just.

This, he knew, was how change truly occurred:

not in clean lines,

not in unanimous shifts,

but in currents — some warm, some cold — learning how to coexist before one finally becomes the climate.

There were early-autumn afternoons when the sky settled into a muted brass hue, soft and steady, even as the wind carried a faint coolness that slipped beneath the warmth like an undercurrent reminding the day that change was coming. He walked across campus on one such afternoon, feeling that duality — warmth holding its ground on the surface, cold gathering its quiet argument beneath it. It was the same atmospheric tension he had begun sensing in the people he encountered.

A group of undergraduates lounged on the grass near the library, laughing about something they'd seen in a nutrition thread online. One of them remarked, with the nonchalance of someone who had never inherited a mythology, "It's wild they ever told people to avoid all fish. It doesn't even make sense chemically."

He heard the sentence float across the lawn — effortless, untroubled, free of the reflexive caution that had shaped entire decades of public messaging. Youth treated the correction as an obvious truth, the way someone born in a renovated house never imagines the previous walls.

He kept walking.

Near the benches beside the old humanities building, he passed two emeritus faculty members in animated conversation. He had known them for decades — thoughtful, seasoned, deeply principled — but their expressions carried the familiar complexity of people navigating a narrative shift not fully their own.

"I still think the guidance was there for a reason," one insisted.

"The chemistry may be more nuanced," the other replied, "but people don't always understand nuance."

"Maybe," came the response, "but changing messaging now... it feels reckless."

Reckless.

That word drifted through the cool air like a leaf that refused to fall. Not malicious, not rigid — just anchored to a time when fear had been easier to standardize than proportion.

He didn't interrupt. They didn't notice him. He continued on, feeling the warm sun on his shoulders but the cool wind along his neck — two layers of temperature coexisting without resolving.

Inside the student center, a different current awaited.

He stepped into the café where a small group of graduate students were gathered around a corner table, laptops open, half-drunk cups of coffee sinking into ring-shaped stains on the wood. Their conversation had that subtle intensity of people analyzing something not because they doubted it, but because they wanted to understand it more deeply.

"...the dataset shows protective equilibrium across almost every demographic," one said.

"And the only outliers are places that never updated the guidance," another added.

"It's not resistance," said a third, "it's lag."

Lag.

Not opposition.

Not refusal.

Just the slow physics of institutional inertia.

He stood for a moment, observing their focus, their ease, the absence of friction in their tone. They were not grappling with the conceptual shift — they were refining it. For them, the correction was not an argument. It was a given.

He stepped back outside, the warm light flickering across the pavement as clouds drifted lazily overhead. He followed the path toward the northern research wing, where the brickwork caught the afternoon sun in soft, tawny patches. A professor stood near the entrance, speaking with a visiting clinician who looked unconvinced in the way people trained in older frameworks often did.

"I'm just not sure the board will be comfortable," the clinician said.

"They'll adjust," the professor replied. "They always do, once the language catches up."

But the clinician shook her head slightly. "It's not the science. It's the habit."

The habit.

He walked past them slowly, and neither noticed him. They were too absorbed in the perennial tug-of-war between what was known and what was felt.

Down the next pathway, he reached the river overlook — a place he visited often, not out of sentiment but because the river offered the kind of continuity that helped him think. The water moved steadily, carrying fallen leaves in long, drifting spirals. Sunlight touched the surface in subtle, shifting bands.

He leaned on the railing and let the breeze move across his face.

Here, away from the conversations and tensions, the truth felt simpler. The river did not care which generation accepted it. The river did not negotiate with habit. It moved forward with the inevitability of things that had already become real.

The world, he knew, was correcting itself — but unevenly.

The young accepted the shift with instinctive ease.

The middle generation approached with cautious recalibration.

The older generation carried the previous era's emotional scaffolding, not out of stubbornness but out of memory.

And he understood — deeply, patiently — that the correction could not flatten these differences. It could only pass through them, season by season, mind by mind.

The wind changed again, slightly cooler now. A sign of the evening approaching.

He exhaled, letting the campus sounds settle behind him. Somewhere inside the buildings, committees debated phrasing; classrooms rehearsed the new framework; students adopted clarity without ever tasting the old confusion.

He turned away from the river and began walking back toward the heart of campus, each step steady, unhurried.

The day was warm.

The wind was cool.

The season was shifting.

And somewhere between the warmth of youth and the coolness of tradition, the truth continued its slow, relentless ascent.

There were mid-autumn mornings when the cold arrived abruptly — a truthful cold, not yet winter's severity but something firmer than the gentle coolness of early fall. The kind of cold that made one inhale more sharply, that made the trees shiver out the last of their leaves, that made the edges of campus feel exposed in a way they hadn't the week before.

He felt that cold now as he crossed the northern footpath. The wind carried a dry rustle of leaves, scraping lightly along the pavement like paper shifting across a wooden desk. The sun was out but dim, filtered through a thin sheet of clouds that made the light feel distant, almost withheld.

He pulled his coat a little tighter and continued walking.

Ahead, the river trail curved toward the sciences complex, and he noticed a familiar scene unfolding: a few early-morning joggers — mostly students — moving along the path with practiced ease. Their breath rose visibly in front of them, but their pace never slowed. Youth rarely flinched at the first chill. They took the new temperature as fact and adjusted without ceremony.

But as he crossed the footbridge, he saw a different figure — an older community member he recognized from public forums, someone outspoken in his lingering concerns. The man walked slowly, hands clasped behind his back, bundled in a heavier coat than the weather yet required. When he saw him, he offered a polite nod, then spoke in the measured tone of someone formulating objections even before voicing them.

"I read another advisory last night," the man said. "Still seems risky to me. Not sure why they're loosening recommendations now. Some things, you just can't be too careful about."

He listened quietly.

The man continued walking beside him, warming to the old rhythm of familiar caution. "Pregnant women shouldn't take chances. We were right to be wary back then. Weren't we?"

The question was rhetorical — a question asked not for clarification but for reassurance.

He answered gently, “Caution is useful when it reflects reality. Less useful when it outlives it.”

The man frowned slightly, as if negotiating the space between habit and understanding. “Maybe. But I still think the old warnings protected people.”

He didn’t argue. He simply nodded, offering the kind of acknowledgment that honors the emotional weight of a long-held belief without affirming the belief itself.

They parted ways near the research wing.

He continued on.

Inside the building, warmth replaced the morning chill. The windows fogged faintly from the temperature difference. Graduate students clustered around tables in the atrium, laptops open, their conversations a low murmur of enthusiasm and precision. He could hear phrases drifting through the space: protective balance, developmental window, nutrient pairing. They spoke with the assured neutrality of people for whom the correction was simply how the world was built.

He paused to watch them — the contrast could not have been sharper. Outside, a man in his seventies clung to the memory of an older narrative. Inside, twenty-year-olds were building entirely new frameworks without ever feeling the friction.

He walked down the hall and passed a door that was slightly ajar. Inside, two mid-career researchers were preparing a presentation for a statewide health summit. Their tone carried the subtle hesitancy of professionals who had lived through the transitional years — younger than the old guard, older than the students.

One said, “We need to be careful how we phrase this. We don’t want the advisory board thinking we’re overturning everything.”

The other replied, “We’re not overturning anything. We’re updating. They’ll resist at first, but the data... the data is where it is.”

He heard the quiet tension in their voices — not fear exactly, but the cautious choreography of people navigating a shifting consensus while keeping one eye on institutional expectations.

He continued walking until he reached a lounge area that overlooked the river. The autumn trees, nearly bare now, revealed more of the water than in previous months. The river looked darker, faster — the seasonal transition advancing with its own kind of inevitability.

He sat for a moment, watching the water move beneath the gray sky. The branches swayed, releasing the last few leaves. A gust of wind rattled the windows.

This, he thought, was the world:

the young moving forward with unencumbered clarity,

the middle negotiating the transition with cautious care,

the old still carrying the emotional residue of another era.

Change was never symmetrical.

Correction was never tidy.

And consensus did not arrive — it emerged.

He rose from the chair, taking one last look at the river, and headed back into the hallway. The building hummed with quiet purpose. Conversations unfolded in rooms large and small. And the truth — the molecular truth he had defended for so long — continued to seep into the world, unevenly but inexorably.

Outside, the wind picked up again.

Cold this time.

But only for now.

He stepped into it without hesitation.

There were late-autumn evenings when the darkness arrived earlier than expected, almost abruptly, as though the day had been edited mid-sentence. The streetlights clicked on before anyone was ready for them, and the remaining warmth in the air retreated faster than the mind could adjust. These were evenings when the world felt momentarily misaligned — the kind of small disorientation that reminded him how transitions always carried traces of the season before.

He walked across the nearly empty campus now, feeling that same disorientation in the conversations he encountered — not chaotic, not contentious, just uneven in the way that weather is uneven at the turning of a season.

He passed a group of undergraduates near the student union, sitting on the low stone wall that edged the walkway. Their breath drifted visibly in the cold as they talked. One of them held up a tablet, reading aloud from an article summarizing updated maternal nutrition guidelines.

A young woman laughed lightly and said, "This makes so much more sense than what my mom always told me."

Her friend replied, "Yeah, our parents got all the warnings, but the chemistry wasn't even lined up back then."

They spoke with the easy certainty of people who had never been burdened by the earlier era's anxieties.

But as he continued walking, he noticed a different tone coming from a nearby bench — two older community members lingering after an alumni event. Their conversation carried the familiar cadence of hesitation.

"It's all changing too fast," one said, arms folded tightly against the cold.

"I don't know," the other replied. "Feels like someone's trying to rewrite the rules."

"But the old rules kept us safe," the first insisted, as though safety and certainty were interchangeable.

He passed them slowly, unnoticed, and felt the duality settle inside him — warm acceptance from one generation, cold resistance from another. The campus reflected this dynamic perfectly: warm light spilling from windows, cold air cutting across the open lawn. Two temperatures coexisting because they must.

He entered the research building, letting the warm air envelope him. The hallways were quiet at this hour, but a few offices still glowed with lamplight. Inside one, a mid-career professor was reviewing a presentation with a younger colleague. Their voices drifted through the open doorway.

“I just worry the advisory board won’t like the tone,” the older one said.

“They’ll adjust,” the younger replied. “They always do after the initial pushback.”

“But they still cling to the old phrasing.”

“So we give them new phrasing that feels familiar.”

He recognized that approach. He had lived inside it for years — adjusting language without diluting truth, offering new clarity in shapes the old could tolerate. It was the quiet diplomacy of scientific transition.

Further down the hall, a classroom door was ajar. Inside, a group of students were finishing a discussion on nutrient interactions. One remarked, half-jokingly, “It’s weird that my grandmother is still terrified of fish.” The others laughed, not unkindly, but with the lightness of people who no longer understood the emotional weight of the old warnings.

He kept walking.

He reached the atrium, where floor-to-ceiling windows overlooked the river. Outside, the last of the daylight clung to the horizon, thinning into a narrow red-gold band before dissolving into deep blue. The river moved slowly now, thickening with cold, its surface beginning to take on the opaque sheen that signaled the first stages of freezing.

He leaned against the railing, watching the water shift under the emerging night. The surface held patches of reflected light from the lampposts — small, luminous fractures in the darkness.

As he watched the river, he felt the generational divide mirror itself in the current:

The surface — slow, dark, heavy — like the older generation holding tightly to what once felt safe.

Below — a steady, invisible movement — like the younger minds carrying the correction forward without hesitation.

Both were real.

Both had weight.

Both were part of the same river.

He stayed there for a long moment, absorbing the layering of it — the cold night, the warm windows, the cautious tones, the confident ones, the friction, the fluency. The correction was moving, yes, but not in a uniform wave. It was moving the way seasons shift:

quietly, unevenly, inevitably.

He stepped back from the railing and began walking toward the exit.

Behind him, the building hummed with light.

Ahead of him, the night settled deeper into the edges of the campus.

Between them — the work continued.

There were early-winter nights when the cold didn't announce itself with wind or snow or spectacle — it simply arrived, settling into the air with a steady, unapologetic confidence. The kind of cold that made the world feel more honest. The kind that stripped away illusion. The kind that reminded him, as it always did, that clarity lived closest to the bare essentials.

He walked through campus under this new cold, the buildings glowing softly against the dark, the windows throwing rectangles of warm, amber light onto the frozen ground. Students moved quickly between buildings, shoulders hunched, their laughter turning to mist in the air. The sidewalks crackled faintly beneath his steps, thin sheets of frost fracturing with each movement.

Every winter carried its own atmosphere.

This one carried a tension he recognized.

As he approached the central promenade, he saw a cluster of graduate students gathered near a lamppost, their voices low but animated. They were discussing a recent paper — a meta-analysis comparing decades of dietary guidance with contemporary biochemical evidence. The conversation was sharp, focused, completely free of the emotional charge that had once surrounded the topic.

“You can see it right here,” one said, pointing to her tablet. “The protective interaction isn’t a fringe idea. It’s foundational.”

Another nodded. “Honestly, it’s wild how long it took to correct the messaging.”

A third added, half-smiling, “Old habits are heavier than data.”

They laughed, not mockingly but with a kind of gentle incredulity — the sound of minds unburdened by the old mythology.

He continued walking, letting their voices dissipate behind him.

As he neared the administrative building, he heard a different conversation — two senior policy advisors stepping briskly through the cold, their tone clipped, their breath rising in short bursts.

"I'm not comfortable endorsing this shift," one said.

"It's not a shift," the other replied. "It's an update."

"Whatever you call it, the public trusts us to keep them safe."

"And keeping them safe means telling them what's actually true."

The first advisor exhaled sharply, the cloud of breath hanging in the cold. "People don't like it when guidance changes. They think it means we were wrong."

"We were incomplete," the second answered plainly. "That's not failure. That's science."

He walked past them unnoticed, feeling the familiar divergence between expectation and understanding. The young accepted the correction as gravity. The middle weighed it against protocol. The older guarded the remnants of the previous narrative, not from stubbornness but from memory.

He felt none of it as conflict.

He felt it as weather.

Inside the library, the warmth enveloped him instantly. He walked through the quiet aisles, passing students huddled over laptops, researchers scribbling notes, a lone faculty member reviewing grant proposals.

At a table near the back, a group of community educators were revising a draft for prenatal outreach materials. Papers were spread across the table, marked with circles, arrows, cross-outs. Their voices were soft, pragmatic.

"I think this section still carries the old tone," one said.

"We need to reframe it," another replied. "Less warning. More explanation."

"But some people will push back."

"They always do. But the next generation won't."

He paused at the end of the row, listening.

One of the educators tapped her pen against a paragraph and said, almost quietly:

"We're not fighting fear. We're replacing it."

Something in that line struck him with the gentle weight of inevitability.

He stepped away, moving toward the far windows overlooking the river. Outside, the water was beginning to freeze along the edges, thin sheets of ice forming delicate patterns like cracked porcelain. The center of the river still flowed freely, dark and calm, a current moving beneath the stiffening surface.

He stood there, studying the contrast — the frozen edges, the flowing core.

It mirrored everything:

The older generation holding to the edges of what they'd been taught.

The younger moving cleanly at the center, unencumbered.

The middle lingering between seasons, negotiating their footing.

The river didn't choose sides.

It simply carried each layer forward.

He remained at the window long enough to watch a thin branch drift past, trapped for a moment in the forming ice before the current pulled it free.

That, too, felt true:

The correction would not force its own acceptance.

It would simply continue moving, and eventually everything would move with it.

He exhaled, watching the fog of his breath touch the glass.

Winter pressed against the edges of the world.

The core kept flowing.

He turned from the window and walked back toward the heart of the library, each step slow, grounded, steady.

The next movement waited, as all movements did — not urgent, not loud, but inevitable.

There were deep-winter afternoons when the daylight felt borrowed — thin, fragile, almost spectral — as though the sun were offering only what it could spare. On afternoons like this, the campus seemed to hold its breath. The buildings hummed. The snow gave off a faint blue sheen. And the cold, sharpened by wind, carried that steady, unyielding truthfulness he had always trusted.

He stepped outside after a long meeting and felt the immediate sting of the air against his face. It wakened something in him — a memory of all the winters he had walked these same paths, carrying the weight of a correction no one else was ready for. Back then, winter felt like the appropriate season for his work. Now, it was simply weather.

As he crossed the quad, he saw a trio of medical residents standing near the entrance of the teaching clinic. They were bundled in coats, their breath rising in pale plumes, but their voices carried a calm confidence.

"...the new study confirms what we've already been teaching," one said.

"It's just consistency at this point," another replied.

"Exactly. It's not controversial anymore."

Their tone was steady, almost relaxed — the language of people who had already moved on from the myth.

But just beyond them, near the bike racks dusted with snow, he noticed an older faculty member speaking with a community volunteer. Their conversation had a different gravity.

"I don't know," the volunteer said. "We told people something else for decades. How do we just... flip that?"

"It's not flipping," the faculty member replied, though his voice lacked conviction. "It's, well... it's complicated."

The volunteer frowned. "Complicated doesn't sell."

And there it was — the old hesitation, the old reflexive protection of fear over nuance, the old idea that complexity was somehow dangerous. He didn't blame them. They were both carrying the weight of an era that had survived by oversimplifying the world.

He walked on.

Inside the main sciences building, warm air fogged his glasses for a moment. Students hurried past, shaking snow from their coats. He turned down the hallway toward the research labs, where he saw a door propped open and heard a spirited discussion inside.

A visiting policy analyst was meeting with a group of researchers. The conversation was nuanced, lively, occasionally tense.

"We need language the agencies won't object to," the analyst said.

"But the agencies are five years behind," a postdoc replied.

"That's why we must tread carefully."

"That's why clarity matters," the postdoc countered.

He paused in the doorway, unnoticed.

The policy analyst rubbed her temples. "The older advisory councils... they're wary. They think changing the narrative undermines trust."

One of the researchers — young, sharp, precise — responded, "Not changing it undermines truth."

The room fell quiet for a moment.

Not hostile.

Not polarized.

Just absorbing.

He stepped back without entering, letting them continue the negotiation between legacy caution and emerging clarity.

Further down the hall, he passed another open room where two students were prepping a presentation for a community workshop. Their slides glowed softly on the wall.

One slide read:

"Understanding Balance: How Nutrients Compete and Protect."

The students were discussing how to explain the concept without triggering defensive reactions from older community members.

"It's the emotional imprint we're working against," one said.

"People remember fear," the other agreed. "But the next generation doesn't. They just see the data."

He walked on, thinking about that.

Fear was an inheritance.

Data was a language.

But clarity — clarity was a temperature shift.

And like all temperature shifts, it moved through the world unevenly.

He reached the end of the hall and stepped into the side stairwell that overlooked the river. Snow had begun again, drifting in slow, diagonal ribbons across the frozen surface. The ice was thick now, opaque and unmoving, but beneath it he knew the current still persisted — not loudly, but relentlessly, reshaping what it touched.

He stood against the cold window, watching the snow settle onto the ice in soft, accumulating layers.

This, too, was how the correction spread:

Layers of understanding falling quietly over time.

Some melted immediately into acceptance.

Some lingered and re-froze into resistance.

And beneath it all, the truth kept moving.

He thought of the older voices he had heard outside — their caution, their unease, their longing for the safety of familiar warnings. He didn't resent them. He understood them. Fear had been their teacher for decades. It did not relinquish its students easily.

But he also thought of the younger voices — their fluency, their ease, their instinctive orientation toward proportion. They did not need convincing. They needed only direction.

Between the two, the middle generation wavered — updating language, negotiating politics, testing the temperature of consensus like someone checking thin ice before stepping forward.

It would take all three circles of weather to finish the season.

He pulled his coat tighter and stepped back into the stairwell.

Winter pressed hard against the glass.

But beneath it — beneath everything — the current flowed on.

There were certain mid-winter nights when the cold settled so deeply into the landscape that even sound seemed to contract, as though the air itself had thickened. On nights like this, the world outside moved slowly — the wind low and deliberate, the trees creaking under the weight of frost, the river muted beneath its solid shell. The campus, usually alive in pockets even after dark, had fallen into a kind of suspended stillness.

He stepped out of the building and felt that stillness immediately.

The sky above was clear, the stars sharp and unmoving. The moon cast a pale sheen across the snow, turning the ground into a vast sheet of cold light. Footprints from earlier in the day had stiffened into crisp impressions; the pathways sparkled faintly under the lamps.

He walked without hurry, breathing in the air that stung just enough to sharpen thought. Winter demanded honesty — from the body, from the mind, from the world. And in nights like these, the divide between generations felt as stark as the temperature shift.

As he crossed the quad, he saw two conversations unfolding in parallel, each lit by a different lamp post, each carrying its own small weather system.

Near the bench by the east entrance, two younger public health fellows were leaving the library, their backpacks slung loosely over their shoulders. Their voices were confident, unencumbered.

"It's obvious once you understand the chemistry," one said.

"Right? I don't even know why the old warnings lasted so long," the other replied.

"They were based on fear."

"They were based on misunderstanding."

"Same thing, sometimes."

They walked on, disappearing into the night with the casual assurance of people who had never inherited the burden of outdated narratives.

But near the opposite lamp post, an older couple — alumni visiting the campus for a winter lecture — were speaking in hushed, concerned tones.

"I just can't reconcile it," the woman said, pulling her scarf tighter. "We were told for decades to avoid certain foods."

"They wouldn't have said it without good reason," the man insisted.

"But now they're saying the opposite."

The man shook his head. “They change their minds too easily. How do we trust that?”

He continued walking, the cold shifting around him like the fault line between two truths lived in different eras.

Inside the medical sciences building, warmth enveloped him — artificial heat humming through vents, a faint scent of coffee lingering from evening study sessions. Down one corridor, a small seminar room was lit brightly. He glanced inside.

A mid-career clinician was leading a training for regional health workers — people old enough to have absorbed the earlier warnings, but young enough to update their practice with measured confidence. Their expressions were thoughtful, attentive.

“...so the goal isn’t to reverse previous guidance,” the clinician said. “The goal is to refine it. Science improves. Our clarity must improve with it.”

One health worker raised his hand. “But some of the older families will push back. They trust what they learned years ago.”

Another added, “It’s not the data they’re resisting. It’s the shift.”

He recognized that, too — the emotional gravity of earlier frameworks.

“They’ll follow if we lead with coherence,” the clinician said. “Not force. Not contradiction. Coherence.”

He moved on.

Further down the hall, near the large windows overlooking the river, a group of undergraduates had gathered around a whiteboard. They were sketching out diagrams in colorful markers, arguing over mechanisms with the exuberance of minds encountering complexity for the first time.

“It’s literally protective,” one said.

“Yeah, but only if the ratio holds,” another corrected.

A third shrugged. “Either way, it’s not scary. It’s elegant.”

Elegant.

Youth had no fear of the truth’s shape.

Only interest.

He walked to the window and stood for a moment, watching the river. The ice near the banks was opaque and still, but further toward the center, faint lines revealed the slow, persistent current beneath. Snow drifted in small spirals across the frozen surface, catching in ridges, settling in layers.

A pattern he knew by heart:

The frozen edges.

The flowing center.

The older generation — holding tight to the cold, to the familiar, to the rules they trusted because they had once required them.

The younger — flowing, steady, unafraid, carrying the correction forward without ever having felt the storm that preceded it.

The middle — standing on the thin surface between those layers, testing the temperature, gauging the strength of the ice before stepping decisively onto the current.

He placed his palm against the glass. It was cold enough that the warmth of his skin fogged the surface in a small, trembling oval.

The truth was like that — warm in its own way, even in the coldest seasons.

He let the fog dissipate, then turned back toward the hallway, where conversations continued in quiet pockets of resistance, acceptance, and transition.

Winter pressed itself into every surface.

But beneath the ice, the current never stopped.

There were late-winter afternoons when the cold no longer felt aggressive, only persistent — not the sharp strike of January, but the steady, patient kind of cold that lingers as though it has negotiated an extension. On afternoons like this, the sky hung low and colorless, a soft gray sheet stretched across the horizon, muting both light and shadow. The world looked flattened, subdued, reflective.

He crossed campus under this muted sky, the snow beneath his feet compacted into a thin, brittle crust that fractured softly with each step. The air carried no wind. Even the trees were still.

It was the sort of day when memory felt closer than usual — not nostalgic, not intrusive, just present. A quiet echo of earlier years when he walked these same paths with a kind of lonely conviction. Back then, he felt as though he were carrying something fragile that the world didn't yet know how to receive.

Now, the fragility was gone. The conviction had migrated outward.

As he approached the biomedical wing, he noticed two figures emerging from the building — both older, both retired faculty members who occasionally returned for guest lectures or advisory panels. They walked slowly, leaning slightly into the cold, their conversation drifting across the quiet space.

"I still don't know if these updates are wise," one murmured.

"We changed the guidelines for a reason," the other replied, his tone hesitant. "What if shifting back confuses people?"

"It's all too fast for my comfort," the first answered. "Too many revisions in too short a span."

He recognized the tone immediately — not opposition, but weariness. A generation fatigued by a world that had rewritten itself multiple times within their career. They weren't resisting the correction. They were resisting the speed of time.

He let them pass.

Inside the building, the air was warm and bright. Posters advertising seminars lined the walls. A few students hurried between rooms, clutching notebooks and tablets. He walked down the hall until he heard voices coming from a medium-sized conference room.

He stopped at the doorway.

Inside, a panel discussion was underway — mid-career clinicians, researchers, and policy advisors gathered around a circular table. Their voices were measured, professional, threaded with the practical tension of people responsible for translating research into real-world policy.

One clinician spoke first:

"The science is solid. The interaction is protective. But I worry about public hesitation."

A policy advisor replied, "It's the older demographic. They're the ones struggling with the shift. Younger families are already there."

A researcher added, "We're not fighting misinformation anymore. We're fighting memory."

He felt that sentence settle into the room — quiet, precise, accurate.

Memory carried its own kind of gravity.

Not scientific.

Not molecular.

But emotional.

He stepped away before anyone noticed him, continuing down the hall.

Further along, he turned a corner and found himself in a smaller lounge area where a group of graduate students sat around a low table, laptops open, coffee cups steaming lightly. Their tone was completely different — fluid, confident, almost lighthearted.

One student said, "We need to emphasize the benefit, not the caution. That's the real message."

Another added, "Exactly. If we keep acting like the old warnings were gospel, we're doing the next generation a disservice."

A third chimed in, smiling, "My mom still panics about it. I told her the body knows what it's doing. She said that sounded 'reckless.'"

They laughed — not at her mother, but at the absurdity of inherited fear.

He stood in the hallway for a moment, noticing how the room glowed with the energy of people who lived outside the emotional residue of earlier decades. They inhabited the correction as naturally as they breathed. They debated implementation, not legitimacy.

Two worlds under one roof.

Two temperatures under one sky.

He stepped outside again, into the quiet cold.

A light snow had begun to fall — not heavy, not dramatic, just a delicate chain of flakes drifting downward in slow, measured spirals. The snow touched the ground lightly at first, dissolving on contact before beginning to accumulate.

He walked toward the river overlook.

The ice on the river had thickened since the last thaw, forming a pale, dull surface with patches of darker shadow beneath. But near the center, a thin seam of open water remained, moving slowly, cutting a narrow line through the frozen sheet.

That seam always found a way.

He watched it for a long moment, feeling the same truth he had felt for years:

progress was a current, not a decree.

the world corrected itself slowly, then suddenly, then slowly again.

generations shifted like weather fronts — warm air, cold air, transitional pockets moving across the same landscape.

The older generation clung to the ice.

The younger flowed at the center.

The middle negotiated the edges.

But all of them — every one of them — were carried forward by the same river.

He took in the scene, the cold settling around him like memory, the snow falling softly, the current moving quietly beneath the surface.

The season had not changed.

But the light had.

And soon the season would follow.

He turned back toward campus, hands in his coat pockets, footprints crisp behind him in the snow.

There were late-winter evenings when the cold didn't deepen so much as settle, as if the season had reached its final expression and was now content to hold its ground. The sky dimmed early, but the darkness felt less like a curtain and more like a soft enclosure. The kind of evening when the world quieted itself without being asked.

He stepped out of the lab building into this dim, enveloping cold. The air tasted metallic. The snow underfoot carried that faint, powdery squeak that only comes in the driest moments of the season. Across campus, lights flickered on in a slow progression; one by one, the buildings illuminated themselves like lanterns aligning along a narrow street.

He adjusted his scarf and began walking toward the central promenade. Students passed him on both sides — brisk, purposeful, untouched by the weight of earlier eras. Their conversations drifted in fragments.

"...so the ratio really matters but not in the way people used to think..."

"...my grandmother refuses to believe it. Says she'll never trust fish again..."

"...it's literally on the NIH site now — why are people still confused?"

"...that's not confusion, that's inertia."

He kept walking.

Ahead, he saw a small gathering outside the lecture hall — people chatting as they exited an evening seminar. Their ages spanned decades, their expressions a mixture of curiosity, discomfort, and faint relief.

A younger attendee, maybe in her early thirties, said, "It's strange thinking about how much fear guided those old recommendations."

An older man beside her replied, “You call it fear. We called it caution.”

“And now?”

He hesitated. “Now I’m... adjusting.”

It was honest.

Hesitation can be integrity when it’s accompanied by movement.

He entered the lecture hall’s lobby just as two professors — both in the latter stages of their careers — walked past him, engaged in a low but intense discussion.

“I don’t oppose the updated guidance,” one said.

“That’s good,” the other replied, “because it’s not optional anymore.”

“It’s not the science I question. It’s the messaging.”

“The messaging is overdue.”

“I know. But people remember what we told them in the nineties. They trust that more than anything we say now.”

The professor paused, then added quietly:

“Fear lingers longer than facts.”

He knew that truth intimately.

He continued down the hallway until he reached a small alcove with floor-to-ceiling windows facing the river. He paused there, letting the cold glass reflect the dim lights behind him. The river outside was a single sheet now — thick, unbroken, pale under the night sky. Only a faint dark line near the center betrayed movement beneath the ice.

He lingered a moment longer before turning back and walking toward the stairwell.

On the lower level, a door to a study room was partly open. He could hear a group of community nutritionists reviewing the new curriculum they were about to teach across rural counties.

One said, "We need to phrase this carefully. Older parents will resist."

Another responded, "It's not resistance. It's loyalty to what they were taught."

A third added, "Well, we're not erasing the past. We're correcting its limitations."

He moved on before they noticed him.

At the far end of the hall, he stepped into the student lounge — an odd mix of warm lighting, humming vending machines, and half-finished project posters taped to the walls.

A handful of undergraduates sat around a large table strewn with notes. Their tone was analytical, but energized.

"It's interesting, isn't it?" one said.

"What is?" another asked.

"How something can be misunderstood for decades because no one questioned the assumptions behind it."

"That's true for a lot of things," someone else replied.

"But this one affects the youngest humans. That's what makes it so important."

Their clarity was neither defiant nor triumphant.

It was simply natural.

They inhabited a world where the correction was self-evident — not because they were rebellious, but because they were unburdened.

He stood unnoticed at the doorway, absorbing the contrast.

Then he stepped outside again.

The snow was falling lightly now — small flakes drifting through the lamplight, turning the air into a luminous haze. The path ahead of him glowed faintly under the thin snow cover, edges softened, footsteps erased.

As he walked, he felt the season reflected in the work:

The older generation, firm and unmoving like the ice;

The younger, like the snow, unfixed and unafraid;

The middle, like the lamplight — illuminating the transition without owning it.

He reached the far edge of campus, where the walkway met the river overlook. He paused there once more, looking down at the frozen surface.

The ice was steady.

The current beneath was steady.

Both were true at the same time.

He exhaled softly, his breath blooming into a faint cloud that drifted upward before dissolving.

The season was holding.

The correction was holding.

And soon, inevitably, the thaw would come.

There were late-winter mornings when the world seemed made of muted silver — the sky a pale wash of diluted light, the snow faintly reflective, the air thin and crystalline. On mornings like this, the horizon felt close, as though distance itself had contracted. The cold was still present, still honest, but it no longer pressed inward. It simply waited.

He stepped outside into this hushed brightness and felt that waiting quality in the air. The buildings around him gleamed with a soft frost, their windows carrying the first hints of the sun. Students moved slowly at this early hour, bundled in coats, their steps deliberate, their voices low.

He walked toward the center of campus, following a path that curved between two large science buildings. Near the entrance of one, he saw a cluster of faculty — mid-career, energetic, still shaking sleep from their eyes — discussing an upcoming regional workshop.

"I think the message is finally getting through," one said, adjusting his backpack.

"To the younger families? Yes," another replied. "To the older communities... we're still seeing hesitation."

"It's the old warnings," a third added. "They had decades to settle. Decades to harden."

"A whole worldview built on a mistake," someone murmured.

He paused as he passed, listening not to the content — he knew every nuance — but to the tone. It carried neither triumph nor frustration. It carried resolve.

Inside the building, warmth enveloped him. A few graduate students were gathered near the first-floor atrium, reviewing a draft of a public health brief. Their conversation was quietly enthusiastic, as though they were crafting something worth believing in.

One said, "If we frame this around fetal development directly, people respond better."

Another nodded. "Mothers especially. They want clarity, not fear."

A third added, "Fear ages badly. Clarity ages well."

He recognized the truth instantly.

Further down the hall, he paused outside a classroom where an early-morning seminar was underway. A professor — thoughtful, methodical — was discussing how scientific corrections disseminate across generations.

"It's not just a matter of evidence," the professor said, pacing slowly. "It's a matter of trust inertia."

A student raised her hand. "Inertia meaning reluctance to update?"

"Reluctance to abandon what once felt protective," the professor clarified.

"So how does the correction spread?" another asked.

“Gradually,” he replied, “and then all at once.”

He almost smiled at that.

He moved on.

Upstairs, in a quiet hallway lined with faculty offices, two community health workers were meeting just outside a door, speaking in soft tones as they adjusted handouts for an upcoming prenatal class.

“I’ll tell them what’s accurate,” one said.

“You’ll get pushback,” the other warned.

“Of course. But pushback isn’t the enemy.”

“What is, then?”

“Stagnation.”

He turned the corner, leaving them to their careful preparations.

As he stepped back outside, the light had strengthened, casting crisp shadows across the snow. The river, visible from between the buildings, showed no sign of movement on its surface — a wide, pale sheet shimmering faintly under the morning sky. But he knew the current persisted beneath, unchanged and continuous.

He walked toward the overlook.

Midway there, he passed two older community members trudging slowly along the path. Their conversation carried that familiar blend of skepticism and lingering caution.

"They're saying the old warnings were exaggerated," one said, his voice tinged with doubt.

"They're changing too much, too fast," the other replied. "Before we know it, they'll say everything was fine all along."

"It wasn't fine."

"No. But it wasn't what we thought."

He felt the weight of their words — not obstruction, but disorientation. A worldview shifting beneath their feet.

He continued toward the river.

At the railing, he stopped and leaned forward slightly, watching the horizon brighten. The ice reflected the sky like brushed metal. A thin dusting of new snow lay atop it, softening the surface, erasing imperfections without hiding the deeper fractures.

Beneath it all, the current moved, steady and indifferent to the season.

He stood there for a long moment, absorbing the layered truth of it:

The older generation, holding to the familiar cold.

The younger, moving easily with the unseen current.

The middle, adjusting the temperature of the narrative one degree at a time.

None of them wrong.

None of them immovable.

All of them part of the same thaw.

He inhaled the cold air, felt it catch at the back of his throat, and exhaled slowly.

Winter had not yet ended.

But the light had shifted.

And light shifts everything.

There were late-winter nights when the cold felt almost ceremonial — not punishing, not sharp, but dignified, as though the season were conducting its own slow exit. The sky held a deep, velvety darkness. The lamps along the walkways cast long, pale halos across the snow, which glittered faintly like powdered glass. Nothing rushed. Even the wind moved with a kind of solemn restraint.

He stepped out into this quiet world, letting the cold settle around him. The buildings rose like dark silhouettes against the sky, their windows glowing softly, each one containing its own small universe of effort — late labs, patient readings, half-empty coffee cups cooling on desks, minds trying to reorder the world one insight at a time.

He began walking toward the west side of campus, where the older brick buildings kept their heat a little less efficiently and their windows fogged more easily. The rhythm of his steps on the hardened snow echoed just enough to remind him of simpler winters long before the science, long before the debates, long before the world had chosen fear over nuance.

As he reached the courtyard near the humanities building, he heard a pair of voices — two mid-career faculty members, bundled against the cold, deep in discussion.

“I gave a talk in Fargo today,” one said.

“How’d it go?”

“Half the room nodded along. The other half looked... lost.”

“Lost how?”

“As though they were being asked to abandon something they’d built their identity around.”

The other sighed. “People invest in warnings. They trust them because they’re simple.”

“And clarity isn’t?”

“Clarity asks more of you.”

He continued on, the truth of that last line lingering in the air behind him.

Further along, near the new biomedical wing, he saw a group of graduate students exiting a late lab session. Their energy was different — sharp, restless, full of possibility. They moved with the easy gait of people who did not fear the correction because they had never feared the myth.

One said, “It’s incredible how much of this was misunderstood for so long.”

Another replied, “Honestly? Not incredible. Just human.”

A third added, “Still — it’s wild that people are just now catching up.”

“Not people,” the first corrected. “Generations.”

They laughed, not dismissively, but with the airy confidence of a cohort unburdened by the old rules.

Inside the building, warmth rose in soft waves. He stepped through the door and heard, from a nearby classroom, a conversation that drew him in with the slightest curiosity. A prenatal educator was rehearsing with a younger colleague — practicing how to guide families through the updated narrative.

The older educator said, “Some of the mothers will cling to the old warnings. It’s not stubbornness. It’s fear.”

The younger replied, “Then we answer fear with proportion.”

“And patience,” the older added.

“And repetition,” the younger concluded.

He paused at the doorway, unnoticed, feeling the lines settle into a kind of inner ledger.

Proportion.

Patience.

Repetition.

They were not merely communication strategies.

They were the architecture of correction.

He wandered onward, down hallways that hummed with quiet machinery and faint fluorescent light. At the end of one corridor, he found a lounge where a few undergraduates were gathered around a table, their laptops open, their coffee cups steaming gently.

One said, “I explained it to my aunt again, and she just stared at me.”

Another replied, “Because she learned it thirty years ago. You learned it yesterday.”

A third added, “You’re not just explaining chemistry. You’re undoing memory.”

He felt something tighten and release in his chest — recognition, not sorrow.

He stepped back outside.

Snow had begun to fall again — slow, deliberate flakes descending through the lamplight, landing softly on the ground. The campus was hushed beneath the snowfall, every sound muffled, every outline softened.

He walked toward the river overlook.

The ice stretched across the water like a pale slate, its surface smoothed by the snowfall, its fractures hidden beneath a thin white layer. But he knew — with the same knowledge that had carried him through decades — that the river underneath was alive, steady, continuous. Unbothered by the hesitation above it.

He leaned on the railing and watched the snowfall drift across the frozen expanse, each flake dissolving silently into the whole.

He thought of the older voices, cautious and reluctant.

He thought of the younger voices, fluent and calm.

He thought of the middle voices, bridging the distance with quiet persistence.

None of them were wrong.

They were simply in different seasons.

The correction was not an argument.

It was a thaw.

And thaws come in layers —

not all at once,

not evenly,

but inevitably.

He stood there until the snowfall thickened and the river seemed to disappear beneath its gathering white.

Then he turned and walked slowly back toward the heart of campus, footprints forming behind him in the new snow — fresh, unmistakable, and leading forward.

There were nights in late winter when the campus felt suspended between seasons — not quite frozen, not quite thawing, but resting in that rare interval where the world pauses, holds its breath, and listens to itself. The lamps across the walkways flickered with a soft, amber steadiness. The snow, thin but persistent, glowed faintly under their light. And the darkness carried a strange gentleness, as though it had agreed to ease its grip.

He stepped into this muted quiet and felt immediately how the air had changed. The cold was still present, but it no longer carried the authority it once did. It felt like a guest taking its leave slowly, politely, unwilling to relinquish the room too abruptly. The season was shifting — not forward, not backward, but inward.

He walked down the path toward the central quad, where a small group of campus staff were finishing their work, packing equipment into a cart. Their voices drifted through the stillness.

One said, “I heard the seminar was packed tonight.”

Another replied, “The new recommendations?”

“Yeah. People are finally getting curious.”

“Curious is good. Curious is where it starts.”

He continued on, the word curious lingering in the quiet air behind him.

Near the old brick auditorium, two older community members stood talking as they prepared to leave a public lecture. Their expressions were thoughtful but uneasy, their breath forming pale clouds in the cold.

“I want to believe it,” one said.

“It’s not about belief,” the other replied. “It’s about what the evidence says.”

“But belief is what I built my decisions on.”

“And evidence is what changes them.”

They paused, neither defensive nor resigned — simply wrestling with the unfamiliar sensation of trust shifting beneath their feet.

He crossed the quad, reached the steps of the newer science building, and stepped inside. The warmth washed over him immediately — the artificial heat, the faint hum of ventilation, the distant buzz of fluorescent lights.

Down the hall, he heard voices from a conference room. He approached quietly.

Inside, a meeting had just concluded. Mid-career researchers, clinicians, and program coordinators were gathering their things, their conversation a mixture of exhaustion and momentum.

"...we need to prepare the rural counties for the new messaging," someone said.

"They're slower to update," another replied.

"That's because their trust structures are older."

"Then we meet them where they are."

"Without surrendering the science."

"Exactly. Accuracy with gentleness."

He lingered just long enough to hear that last phrase — accuracy with gentleness — before moving on.

Further down the hall, he passed a study nook where two students sat reviewing lecture notes, their voices low but certain.

"I don't get why it was misunderstood for so long," one said.

"People were scared," the other replied.

"But the data..."

"The data wasn't the problem."

"What was?"

"The story they told about it."

He slowed his pace, letting that truth arrive fully:

facts change the mind,

stories change the behavior.

He walked on.

At the end of the building, he stepped through a set of glass doors that opened to a small courtyard overlooking the river. The night air cooled his face instantly. The courtyard stones were dusted with a thin layer of snow, and the bare trees cast delicate, latticed shadows across the ground.

He moved toward the railing overlooking the frozen river.

The ice was subtly different now — still thick, still pale, still holding the weight of winter, but its edges appeared softened, slightly dulled, as though the season were letting go of its rigidity in increments too small to measure. The faintest suggestion of melt glimmered near the banks, a thin, reflective sheen that caught the lamplight.

He watched it quietly.

The older generation, he thought, was like the ice — steady, protective, shaped by a season that once demanded vigilance. Their caution wasn't defiance; it was history retaining its form.

The younger generation was like the sky above — open, expanding, lit with the possibility of change. They didn't fear the correction because they weren't shaped by the storm that preceded it.

And the middle generation — policymakers, clinicians, educators — stood exactly where he now stood: facing the river, reading its surface, sensing the shift, negotiating the narrative between what had been frozen and what was beginning to flow.

He breathed out slowly.

The air carried the faint scent of cold water held in suspension.

The snow continued falling lightly, each flake dissolving into the larger silence.

Winter had not relinquished its hold, but it had conceded its inevitability.

He stayed there for a long moment, letting the stillness of the landscape settle into him — the river, the ice, the soft, unresolved night.

Then he turned back toward the campus, the quiet crunch of his footsteps marking his passage through a season that was already beginning to yield.

There were late-winter afternoons when the light behaved strangely — not bright, not dim, but diffused, as though the sun were hidden behind multiple layers of sheer cloth. The snow reflected this muted light with a faint pearl sheen. Footsteps echoed differently in this atmosphere, softer, as if the world had decided to speak in a lower tone.

He walked across campus under that softened light, feeling the shift in temperature — not warmer, not yet, but less absolute. The cold had lost its authority. It persisted only because winter had momentum.

Near the main science building, he saw a group of graduate assistants gathered around a portable heater, reviewing materials for an outreach lecture scheduled in a rural community two hours away. Their tone was pragmatic, focused.

One said, “We have to be careful with the phrasing.”

Another added, “They still trust the old advisories.”

A third replied, “Then we frame it as continuity, not contradiction.”

“Continuity of what?”

“Clarity,” the third answered. “Clarity that took twenty years to refine.”

He watched them for a moment — young scientists preparing to enter rooms where stories were older than data. They didn’t seem intimidated. They seemed ready.

He continued walking.

Inside the main atrium, warmth rose from the building’s central vents, carrying the scent of coffee and the faint static crackle of winter clothing. A few undergraduate students were huddled around a table, practicing for a panel discussion.

One said, “We’re not saying the old guidelines were wrong. We’re saying they were incomplete.”

Another corrected him gently, “We’re saying they were shaped by fear, not proportion.”

A third added, “Fear is easy to inherit. Proportion you have to learn.”

He almost paused to write that line down — not because it was profound, but because it was accurate.

Farther down the hallway, he approached a small lounge where two older faculty members sat by the window, speaking quietly over cups of tea. There was something solemn in their posture, as though they were carrying the weight of decades not just in knowledge, but in responsibility.

One said, "I remember when the advisory first came out. We felt... righteous."

The other nodded. "We believed we were protecting people."

"We were."

"For a moment," the first corrected. "Then the moment changed."

"And we did not."

He moved past, feeling both the honesty and the ache of those words.

Upstairs, in a narrow corridor lined with posters from past conferences, he heard the low hum of conversation coming from a seminar room. A dozen community health educators were gathered around a whiteboard, discussing updated materials for clinics across the state.

"It's going to take years," one said.

"Generational cycles," another replied.

"Will we see the full shift?" a third asked.

"Maybe not," the instructor answered. "But they will."

He continued down the hall and stepped into the older wing of the building — the part that still carried the faint scent of chalk dust and varnished wood. A single office light was on. Inside, a researcher sat at her desk, speaking on a video call.

"...yes, I understand the hesitation," she said calmly. "But the biochemical dynamics are not a matter of belief. They are measurable. They are reproducible. And they have been misunderstood for decades."

She paused, listening.

"Your patients will be frightened," she continued. "That is normal. Fear ages faster than evidence. Work with it, not against it."

He stepped away, letting the door fall silent behind him.

Outside once more, he walked toward the river overlook. The path was lightly dusted with new snow, and his footprints appeared crisp and distinct behind him. The sky above had taken on a faint lavender hue — one of those rare winter colors that signaled the approach of evening even before the sun touched the horizon.

At the railing, he paused.

The river was still a hard, flat expanse — but the ice was subtly changing. Fine cracks spidered across its surface, not dangerous yet, but inevitable. Near the center, the dark seam of water had widened just slightly, revealing the quiet persistence of the current beneath.

He watched it closely, the way one watches the beginning of a season shift.

The older worldview was the thick ice — firm, protective, slow to shift.

The younger worldview was the open seam — narrow, certain, alive with movement.

And the middle — the communicators, the clinicians, the educators — were the faint cracks bridging the two, carrying pressure from both sides, shaping the thaw that would come.

He inhaled the cold air and exhaled slowly.

Truth doesn't rush.

It accumulates.

He turned from the railing, the lavender light deepening around him, and began walking back toward the building, the snow whispering under each step.

There were late-season evenings when the air felt exquisitely thin — not cold enough to sting, not warm enough to comfort, but balanced at a precise point between endurance and release. The sky above stretched in a pale gradient of fading blues, the horizon softening into violet as the last traces of daylight withdrew. You could sense the change before you could see it. The atmosphere carried the quiet anticipation of something about to shift.

He stepped out of the building and into this delicate equilibrium. The world seemed muted, not asleep but contemplative. The snow on the ground had thinned to a brittle crust along the edges of the walkways, and patches of pavement showed through like islands in a receding tide. The lamps along the path flickered on with a faint hum, casting elongated shadows that wavered slightly with the movement of the air.

He began walking without urgency, following the curved path toward the center of campus. The evening was alive with small pockets of conversation — subdued, thoughtful, unhurried.

Near the main entrance of the wellness center, he passed two younger faculty members speaking in soft, reflective tones.

"...honestly, I never realized how much fear shaped the old guidance," one said.

"It wasn't fear at first," the other replied. "It became fear over time."

"How?"

"When caution hardens into doctrine. When doctrine stops questioning itself."

He slowed for only a moment before moving on, leaving their voices to dissolve into the air behind him.

Farther along, near the benches overlooking the quad, he noticed an older couple sitting side by side. They wore heavy coats and thick gloves, their posture suggesting a long conversation rather than a short one. Their voices drifted toward him — familiar, earnest, tinged with the weight of lived experience.

"I just can't understand why they didn't tell us this earlier," the woman said.

"They didn't know," the man replied gently.

"They acted like they did."

"They acted like they believed they were protecting us."

"And now... what do we do with that?"

"We learn what we can. And we keep going."

He continued walking, absorbing the tenderness in their quiet exchange — not resentment, not defiance, but a slow, steady recalibration of trust.

Inside the science building, warmth embraced him. The hallways glowed with soft, artificial light. Down one corridor, he saw a small group of public health students rehearsing for a community forum.

One said, "Don't say the old way was wrong. Say the new way is clearer."

Another nodded. "People accept clarity. They resist contradiction."

A third added, "Fear is a habit. Clarity is a practice."

He paused at that last line — a kind of internal punctuation that settled neatly into the rhythm of the work.

He moved deeper into the building.

From a nearby classroom, he heard the tail end of a faculty discussion.

"...the older generation lived the warning, not the mechanism," someone said.

"That's why the correction feels like a reversal to them," another answered.

"It isn't a reversal."

"No. It's a refinement."

"And refinements feel like betrayals when you've anchored yourself to a simpler story."

The room fell briefly silent before someone added quietly:

"Science outlives the stories we tell about it."

He stepped away before the silence resolved.

At the end of the hall, he pushed open the side door and walked out into the cooling air. The sky had darkened slightly, deepening into a rich indigo. A thin breeze moved through the trees, carrying with it the faint scent of thawing branches and damp earth beginning to wake beneath the frozen ground.

He followed the familiar path toward the river overlook.

As he approached, he saw the ice again — pale, wide, unwavering — but now, subtle changes had begun to appear. The fractures along the edges had grown more pronounced. A faint darkening near the center hinted at the widening seam beneath. The surface still held its shape, but the season beneath was in motion.

He leaned on the railing and watched the river breathe through its constraints.

The older worldview was the frozen surface — strong, still, protective.

The younger worldview was the widening seam — fluid, certain, forward-moving.

And the middle — the educators, scientists, communicators — were the faint cracks that let the future in.

It was not conflict.

It was sequence.

He inhaled the evening air — cool, thin, balanced — and exhaled slowly as the horizon continued to darken.

The season had not changed.

But the season was preparing to.

He turned from the overlook, the lamps flickering softly behind him, and walked back toward campus under the quiet, patient sky.

There were evenings—thin, windless, and strangely luminous—when the entire campus seemed to balance on a single breath. The sky above carried a faint, powdery glow, the kind that comes not from daylight but from snow reflecting the last traces of twilight. Everything felt lightly suspended. Even time seemed to hesitate, as if choosing whether to lean toward winter or toward whatever came next.

He stepped into that suspended quiet with the ease of someone who had learned to read the subtle language of seasons. The path ahead was mostly clear now, edged by shallow ridges of old snow that had melted and refrozen into rough, translucent borders. His footsteps tapped lightly against the pavement, the sound crisp but subdued, merging with the stillness rather than breaking it.

As he passed the older lecture hall, he noticed two retired professors leaving through the side doors, their scarves pulled tight, their movements deliberate. Their conversation drifted toward him on the soft, evening air.

"...the data has been there for years," one said, his voice tinged with a resigned perplexity.

"But the story took longer to adapt," the other replied.

"It shouldn't have."

"It couldn't have," the second corrected gently. "People don't update what they've trusted for decades. Not easily."

"And now we ask them to?"

"Now we give them room to."

He passed them with a quiet nod, feeling the sincerity behind their words. They were not resisting the correction; they were grieving the time it took to reach it.

Farther along, on a bench overlooking the quad, two younger researchers huddled over a tablet, reviewing slides for an upcoming symposium. Their tone carried none of the older generation's hesitation.

One said, "It's incredible how clean the protective interaction looks when you model it correctly."

The other nodded. "It's elegant. Almost too elegant for how messy the communication has been."

"That's why our generation gets it faster," the first added. "We weren't molded by the warnings."

"We weren't molded by the fear," the other corrected.

"Fear is a mold," the first said. "Clarity is a solvent."

He let their voices fade as he continued toward the biomedical wing.

Inside, he found a quiet hum of activity—graduate students at whiteboards, researchers carrying notebooks, a few early-career clinicians preparing materials for the next day's rounds. The atmosphere was determined, but not tense. It felt like a place that had accepted its role in a long correction and was moving with deliberate precision.

Near one corner of the atrium, a pair of community educators were rehearsing how to talk to expectant mothers at a regional clinic.

One said, "We focus on development, not danger."

"Right," the other replied. "We describe how things work, not just what to avoid."

"And we say it calmly."

"And consistently."

"And without condescension."

"Especially without condescension."

Their voices held a kind of gentle courage—a recognition that clarity must arrive quietly to be accepted.

He left the building and walked toward the library, where warm, amber light shone through tall windows. Inside, a late-night study group was gathered, their coats draped over chairs, their notebooks spread out in overlapping layers.

He paused near the doorway, listening.

One student said, "It's not that the old warnings were malicious."

Another shook her head. “No. They were protective... but incomplete.”

A third added softly, “Incomplete guidance ages like fear.”

“And updated guidance ages like reason,” someone else said.

They all nodded, as though acknowledging a truth so familiar it no longer sparked debate.

He stepped outside again, toward the river path.

The air had cooled further, but the cold now felt shallow—less structural, more cosmetic. Snowflakes drifted slowly downward, sparse enough to appear individually, each one catching light briefly before disappearing. The kind of snowfall that signals neither storm nor thaw but the quiet in between.

He approached the overlook.

The river below was still encased in ice, but the surface was subtly different tonight. New fractures had begun to appear—hairline fissures radiating outward in quiet, delicate lines. They weren’t dangerous yet. But they were honest.

He stood there as the evening settled into full darkness, watching the faint glimmer of the river’s hidden movement beneath the rigid surface.

The older generation remained the ice—structured, certain, shaped by memory.

The younger remained the current—fluid, confident, shaped by proportion.

And the middle remained the fractures—subtle, necessary, and quietly transformative.

No one was right or wrong.

They were simply in different stages of thaw.

He exhaled, his breath forming a small cloud that dissolved almost immediately.

The season was preparing to yield.

So was the world.

He turned from the railing and began walking back toward the warm glow of the campus, footprints forming behind him in soft, deliberate intervals.

There were evenings near the end of winter when the world felt almost overexposed—not in brightness, but in honesty. The landscape revealed itself without ornament: the bare trees, the thinning snow, the muted edges of buildings that had endured months of cold. Nothing concealed itself. Nothing pretended to be more than it was. It was a season stripped to essentials.

He stepped out into this clear, unadorned night and felt the same unvarnished quality in the air. The temperature hovered just below freezing—the kind of cold that didn't bite but reminded you it could if it chose to. The lamps along the walkway cast gentle halos across the ground, turning the pavement into a sequence of soft circles that guided his steps.

He walked toward the eastern quad, where the last traces of students were leaving the science buildings. A pair of them lingered near the entrance, speaking in quiet but animated tones.

"It's strange," one said, adjusting her backpack. "My mom still sends me articles warning about it."

"That's because fear stays in circulation longer than fact," the other replied.

"She trusts the old story."

"Stories don't retire. They fade. Slowly."

He continued on, the truth of that last line echoing in the stillness behind him.

Near the library steps, a midcareer clinician spoke with a younger colleague as they left a faculty forum.

"I think the correction is finally getting traction," the younger said.

"Among your cohort, yes," the older replied.

"And yours?"

"We're trying."

"What slows it down?"

"Responsibility."

"To what?"

"To everything we once told people in good faith."

He understood that. He had lived inside that very tension.

He entered the library for a moment, letting the warmth greet him. The air inside carried the faint scent of books, dust warmed by lamplight, and the quiet murmur of pages turning. Near a long table, a group of graduate researchers were reviewing a draft of an upcoming publication.

One said, “The evidence is clear. The mechanism is clear.”

Another nodded. “Then what’s the obstacle?”

“The public’s muscle memory.”

“Can science overcome muscle memory?”

Someone answered softly, “Only if it’s patient enough.”

He stepped away, letting that sentence become part of the room’s quiet hum.

Outside again, he crossed the walkway toward the humanities wing. There, on a bench under a flickering lamp, sat two older community members who had just left an evening outreach event. They spoke with the unguarded candor of people sorting through something that unsettled them.

“I trusted the old warnings,” the woman said, her gloves clasped tightly.

“So did everyone,” the man replied.

“But now we’re told it was incomplete.”

“It was.”

“Why didn’t they know earlier?”

“They were looking at the wrong danger.”

“And now?”

“Now they’re looking at the right one.”

She shook her head slowly, not in disagreement, but in the slow rhythm of adjustment.

He moved past them quietly, letting their uncertainty fold into the gentle darkness of the evening.

The air carried the subtle scent of thawing earth. Not visible yet, not audible yet, but present—an undercurrent rising through the cold.

He followed the familiar path toward the river.

As he approached the overlook, he felt the temperature drop slightly. The railing was cold under his hand, the metal stiff and unyielding. Below, the river remained a wide, pale sheet of ice—but now, the fractures were more prominent, mapping themselves across the surface like a faint, silvery network.

The fissures were delicate but persistent.

And the seam of open water near the center had widened by a few inches, just enough to reveal a deeper darkness beneath.

He watched the river for a long time, letting its quiet geometry sink into him.

The older generation—the ice—still held its form.

The younger generation—the current—still moved freely beneath.

And the middle generation—the fractures—did the work of transition, distributing pressure, inch by inch, degree by degree.

It was not dramatic.

It was not fast.

It was not even visible to most.

But it was happening.

He breathed deeply, letting the cold settle into his lungs before exhaling slowly into the night.

The thaw had not begun.

But the world was preparing for it.

He turned away from the river and began walking back toward the quiet glow of the campus, each step steady, deliberate, unhurried.

There were nights at the tail end of winter when the world lay so still that even small sounds seemed amplified—a door closing, a distant car passing on the far edge of campus, the soft crackle of frost shifting beneath the surface of the snow. It was a quiet not of emptiness, but of anticipation, as though the landscape itself knew it was on the cusp of change.

He stepped into that quiet with a sense of recognition. Winter had settled into its final shape. The cold remained, but its character had softened; it no longer enforced itself, it merely lingered. The lamps along the main walkway glowed with a calm, golden steadiness, their halos diffusing into the light snow that drifted through the air.

He walked toward the research quad, where he noticed a familiar scene—clusters of conversations, each one carrying its own temperature, its own season, its own pace of adaptation.

Near the entrance to the long-standing physiology building, he spotted two community health educators finishing a discussion after a late training session.

"...they're not resisting the science," one said, pulling her coat tighter.

"They're resisting the idea that they were misled," the other replied.

"We're not saying they were misled."

"They hear it that way."

"Well, then we need to say it differently."

"We've been saying it differently for years."

"Then we keep going."

Their voices drifted behind him, shaped not by frustration but by endurance.

A few steps further, perched on a bench under a lamp that flickered slightly with the evening breeze, sat two younger graduate students reviewing notes for an upcoming conference presentation.

"It's wild," one said, "how clean the protective mechanism looks in the data. It's almost... elegant."

The other nodded. "But the messaging has to stay grounded. People don't trust elegant answers."

"Why not?"

"Because fear never arrives elegantly."

He walked past, a faint smile tugging at the corner of his mouth. Their clarity was refreshing—direct, proportional, unburdened.

Inside the newer biomedical building, warmth met him in a gentle wave. He walked through the quiet hallway lined with framed publications, each one bearing the names of researchers who had contributed to the slow, patient architecture of truth.

From an office with its door partly ajar, he overheard two mid-career scientists discussing the latest batch of review feedback.

“The reviewers liked the data,” one said.

“They always like the data.”

“But they flagged the language.”

“Of course they did.”

“They want it ‘more cautious.’”

The other sighed. “...we’ve been cautious for twenty years.”

“Too cautious.”

“No. Just cautious enough to survive the politics.”

“And now?”

“Now they want cautious clarity.”

“That’s contradictory.”

“It’s transitional.”

He stepped away, leaving their soft laughter behind him.

A few doors down, a student study group gathered near a whiteboard. Their voices carried a different kind of energy—steady, curious, alive with the certainty of a generation that didn’t have to unlearn anything.

One student said, "My professor said the biggest obstacle isn't evidence—it's emotional residue."

Another replied, "Yeah. People don't cling to facts. They cling to the feelings facts gave them."

A third added, "Then our job is to give them new feelings."

Someone else said quietly, "No... our job is to give them proportion."

He lingered just long enough to let that truth settle inside him.

Back outside, he felt the cold shift—lighter now, moving through the air with the restraint of a season losing its authority. He followed the familiar path toward the river, his footsteps crisp on the thin crust of snow.

At the overlook, he rested his hands on the railing.

The river was still iced over, but the surface carried the unmistakable signs of approaching change. The network of fractures had expanded, feeding into one another, distributing tension in delicate, branching lines. The open seam near the center had widened another inch—small, nearly invisible at a distance, but significant to anyone who understood how thaws begin.

He watched it, absorbing the quiet geometry of the moment.

The older generation—the solid sheet of ice—held to its form with quiet dignity.

The younger generation—the dark seam of open water—moved freely beneath.

And the middle—the branching fractures—translated pressure into progress.

No conflict.

Only sequence.

Only season.

He breathed in the faint scent of cold water pushing upward beneath the ice, a reminder that the current had never stopped—not once, not for an instant—even when the surface appeared still.

He exhaled slowly, letting the breath drift into the delicate snowfall.

The world had not changed.

It was changing.

And that distinction mattered.

He turned from the railing and began the slow walk back toward the heart of campus, the lamps glowing softly, the snow drifting gently in the quiet air, and the season shifting by degrees.

There were late-winter nights when the landscape felt both exhausted and alert, as though the season itself had reached the edge of its endurance. The air was still cold, unmistakably cold, but it no longer carried conviction. It clung to the world out of habit. The sky above was a muted gradient—deep blue pressed gently into grey, the horizon holding a faint trace of saffron that seemed to belong to a different season entirely.

He stepped outside into that paradox of a night. The walkways were mostly clear now, but thin sheets of frost clung to their edges like the last remnants of a doctrine that had not yet realized it was obsolete. His breath formed pale clouds before dissolving quickly into the open air, as if even the cold was tired of itself.

He followed the main path toward the center of campus, where conversations floated like small weather systems drifting across the evening.

Near the illuminated entrance of the student union, two younger faculty members lingered after an interdisciplinary panel. Their voices carried the calm certainty of people who no longer regarded the correction as a controversy.

"...the mechanism is stable, reproducible, well-documented," one said.

"The only instability is in public perception," the other replied.

"That's generational."

"That's emotional."

"That's the same thing."

He walked on, leaving their voices to settle into the gentle hum of the building.

Farther along, near a bike rack dusted with frost, an older couple stood beneath a lamp, their coats zipped high, their posture slightly hunched against the lingering chill. Their conversation was quieter, more tentative.

"I believed the old warnings because they were simple," the woman said.

"We all did," the man replied.

"But now they're saying it was... never that simple."

"It never is."

She looked down at the ground. "Why do I feel like I followed the wrong map?"

"You followed the best map we had," he said. "Now we have a better one."

He continued walking, absorbing the quiet dignity in their exchange—a willingness to shift, even late, even with uncertainty.

Inside the biomedical building, the warmth greeted him in a soft rush. The hallways buzzed with low conversation and the rustling of jackets. Students and researchers passed him with notebooks tucked under their arms, eyes bright despite the late hour.

He paused near a seminar room where a mid-career scientist and a health policy advisor were reviewing the draft of an upcoming report.

"It's not that people distrust the science," the scientist said.

"No," the advisor replied. "They distrust how often the guidance changes."

"But that's what science does—refine, update, calibrate."

"And yet to the public, refining looks like reversing."

"Then we teach them the difference."

"We've been trying."

"Then we keep trying."

He moved on, letting the cadence of their persistence settle behind him.

Upstairs, in a smaller lounge illuminated by the soft glow of floor lamps, a group of graduate students sat around a table, their laptops open, their conversation circling the complexities of communication rather than the science itself.

One said, “It’s fascinating—fear scales quickly.”

Another added, “Clarity doesn’t. It grows slowly.”

A third looked up from her screen and said, “Then our job is to grow it carefully.”

He paused at the doorway long enough to see how naturally they carried the correction, how effortlessly they navigated what once felt like an insurmountable cultural barrier.

Outside again, he felt the temperature dip slightly, a reminder that winter would not depart without a few final gestures. He followed the familiar path toward the river overlook, the lamps casting elongated shadows across the thinning snow.

At the railing, he paused.

The river was still frozen, but the transitions were unmistakable now. The fractures across the ice had grown into delicate networks of intersecting lines, each one carrying a whisper of the pressure beneath. The dark seam in the center had widened yet again, revealing more of the moving water below—slow, steady, certain.

He watched the river in silence.

The older generation—the ice—held its structure because it had learned to survive by holding.

The younger generation—the current—moved without hesitation, because it had never known anything else.

And the middle generation—the fractures—did the subtle work that neither side could: translating pressure into possibility.

He let that thought rest in the quiet space between breaths.

The night air brushed against his face, cold but soft.

The river murmured beneath its frozen shell.

The lamps flickered gently behind him.

The thaw had not begun, not truly.

But the world was positioned for it.

Aligned for it.

Ready for it.

He turned from the river and began walking back toward the warm lights of campus, each step deliberate, steady, as the season—not yet changing, but preparing to—settled around him.

There were nights so close to spring that winter seemed to hover in place, unwilling to retreat yet no longer capable of asserting itself. The air held that unmistakable ambiguity — not cold, not warm, but suspended somewhere between conviction and surrender. The sky above carried a diluted softness, as though the season had been thinned by its own endurance. It was the kind of night where even silence felt transitional.

He stepped into that in-between air and sensed immediately how the world had changed. Not dramatically. Not visibly. But quietly — the way a long-held belief loosens its grip, not because it is forced, but because the mind has finally grown tired of holding it so tightly.

The walkways gleamed faintly beneath a film of frost. His steps made a muted sound, softer than snow, sharper than bare pavement — a sound that belonged only to the thinning edge of a season.

Ahead, he noticed a small group leaving the auditorium after an evening seminar. Their coats were pulled close, their breath visible in the dim light, but their conversation carried warmth.

One of the mid-career researchers said, “The younger audience asked all the right questions tonight.”

A colleague nodded. “Because they weren’t burdened by the old anxieties.”

“What about the older attendees?”

“They listened,” the colleague said. “And they didn’t challenge. That’s its own kind of progress.”

“It’s slow.”

“It’s real.”

He passed them quietly, the cadence of their words settling like the soft frost beneath his feet.

Further along, near a row of bike racks half-buried in old snow, two older community members stood speaking in murmurs, their tones carrying a mix of uncertainty and contemplation.

"I always thought avoiding certain fish was the safest thing," the woman said.

"It felt safe," the man replied.

"And now they say it kept us from the nutrients we needed."

"Not intentionally."

"No... but still."

He paused before adding, "It takes time to let go of fear that tried to protect you."

He walked past them slowly, letting the quiet bravery of their conversation linger behind him.

Inside the biomedical building, warmth met him once more. Down the main hallway, a late-night study group had gathered around a glowing laptop. Their voices carried the tone of people who considered clarity not an achievement but an expectation.

One said, "The interaction isn't complicated. The communication was."

Another replied, "Because fear was easier than nuance."

A third added, "Fear is fast. Science is slow."

"And corrections," someone else said softly, "are slower."

He moved on, stopping near the stairwell where he overheard two faculty members — both experienced, both measured — discussing upcoming workshops for regional clinics.

“We have to speak gently,” one said.

“We have been,” the other replied.

“It still feels like we’re asking them to abandon something essential.”

“We’re asking them to trust something new.”

“That’s harder.”

“That’s necessary.”

Their voices drifted into the stairwell as he descended toward the lower exit.

Outside again, the atmosphere felt subtly different — the cold thinner, the air carrying a faint scent of damp earth beginning to push upward through the frozen ground. He walked toward the river path, his footfalls steady, the lamps along the way flickering with the early signs of seasonal instability.

At the overlook, he paused.

The river below remained encased in ice, but it no longer looked solid. Fine shards of meltwater shimmered beneath the surface. The web of fractures had grown more intricate, forming delicate, branching pathways across the ice like the faint lines of an old map. And at the very center, the seam of open water had widened — not enough for anyone else to notice, but enough for him to recognize the truth:

The thaw was no longer a future event.

It was a current one.

Quiet.

Measured.

Undeniable.

The older generation — the ice — still held its shape with dignity.

The younger generation — the seam — flowed with untroubled certainty.

The middle — the fractures — carried the tension between them with grace.

It was not conflict.

It was choreography.

He rested both hands on the cold railing, feeling the faint vibration of the hidden current beneath the surface.

The world had not declared its change.

It had committed to it.

He breathed in deeply, letting the dampness of early thaw fill his lungs, then exhaled slowly into the soft evening air.

Winter was still present.

But spring had begun its quiet work.

He turned from the river and walked back toward the campus lights — slow, steady, and certain — as the world shifted by degrees around him.

There were nights just before the thaw when the cold felt like a memory of itself — present, but dimmed, as though winter were repeating its final lines out of obligation rather than conviction. The sky held a faint luminescence that did not come from the moon but from the atmosphere itself, a soft brightness diffused through thin clouds. It was the kind of light that made everything appear suspended: the buildings, the bare trees, even the air.

He stepped outside and sensed the shift immediately. It wasn't warmth. It wasn't relief. It was the quiet recognition that the season had passed its peak. The snow beneath his feet had grown granular, its edges softened by days hovering near freezing. The walkways glistened faintly. The lamps cast their halos farther across the damp pavement.

He walked toward the northern quad, where a late meeting in the science building had just concluded. Three researchers emerged from the doors, their coats open despite the cold, their conversation lingering in that reflective space between work and contemplation.

One said, "The room didn't push back tonight."

"Not even the older attendees?" another asked.

"No. They were quiet."

"Quiet is good," the third murmured. "Quiet means the shift has begun."

"It means," the first replied, "that resistance has grown tired."

He moved past them, their words settling into the soft air behind him.

Near the bench by the frozen fountain, he noticed an older woman sitting alone, hands folded in her lap, scarf pulled snug around her neck. She was reading a pamphlet from the lecture, turning it slowly in her hands. As he approached, he heard her speaking softly to the man beside her — her husband, perhaps — who sat with his elbows on his knees, listening intently.

She said, "I thought I understood. I really did."

He answered gently, "You understood what they taught us."

"But they're saying it was... incomplete."

"It was the best they knew at the time."

She closed the pamphlet. "I don't like changing my mind."

He rested a hand on hers. "Most people don't. But you're trying."

He walked on, feeling the quiet bravery in their conversation. It wasn't acceptance yet, but it was orientation — a beginning.

Inside the biomedical building, the warmth brushed against him, carrying the faint hum of late-night research. Down the hallway, he heard a group of younger scientists discussing a pilot program for rural clinics.

"We're not imposing anything," one said.

"We're offering clarity," another added.

"And we're doing it gently," someone else insisted.

"Gently," the leader agreed, "but steadily."

He paused near the doorway long enough to feel the conviction in their tone — not forceful, not urgent, but certain.

A few steps later, he passed a glass-walled study room where two students sat at a whiteboard covered in diagrams. Their conversation flowed with the easy confidence of those who no longer felt the emotional residue of earlier decades.

One said, “To us, it’s obvious.”

“It is now,” the other replied.

“It will be to them, too.”

“In time.”

“In proportion,” the first corrected, smiling.

He continued down the hall and exited through a side door.

Outside, he breathed in air that carried the faintest scent of thawing soil — not obvious, not strong, but unmistakable to someone who had walked these grounds through many seasons. The sky had darkened into a soft navy. The lamps flickered with the gentle instability that comes from moisture rising through the cold.

He followed the familiar path to the river.

When he reached the overlook, he rested his hands on the railing — the metal cold but no longer biting — and looked down at the water below.

The river had changed.

The ice was still present, but its authority was fading. The fractures were more pronounced now, branching like the veins of a leaf. Small pools of meltwater had formed on the surface, glistening under the lamps. The seam of open water in the center had widened visibly — a dark ribbon cutting through the pale surface, the current beneath moving with quiet determination.

He watched it for a long moment.

The older generation — the ice — still held its form, but it was thinning.

The younger generation — the current — flowed openly now, no longer hidden.

And the middle generation — the fractures — carried the delicate work of translating tension into motion.

It was not conflict.

It was not friction.

It was the natural choreography of change.

The world was not rejecting what it once believed.

It was outgrowing it.

He breathed in deeply, the air cool but gentler than it had been in months.

Winter remained.

But the thaw had committed itself.

He watched the river shift, quiet and inevitable beneath the night sky, then turned and began walking back toward the softly glowing campus, his pace steady in the hush of the coming season.

There were nights, just at the threshold of seasonal change, when the air felt as if it were listening — not observing, not reacting, but listening in the way a still room listens after a profound truth has been spoken. The temperature held itself delicately, neither cold nor warm, as though refusing to declare allegiance to the season preparing to arrive.

He stepped out into that listening air.

The walkways gleamed with a damp sheen, reflecting the faint gold of the lamps overhead. The snowpacks had eroded into soft, uneven mounds, their edges blurred, as if winter were slowly releasing its hold piece by piece. A few remnants of ice clung to the pavement in translucent patches, catching the light like fragments of old glass.

He walked toward the central promenade.

Ahead, two younger faculty members were leaving the public outreach center, their conversation carrying an almost philosophical tone.

"...the older audience didn't challenge it tonight," one said.

"Because the conflict wasn't about the science," the other replied.

"No."

"It was about the fear of admitting the world changed without asking for their permission."

"That's a hard truth."

"That's why it needs a soft arrival."

He continued past them, feeling the resonance of those last words — soft arrival — settle gently into the evening.

Farther along, at the bench under the lamppost where the snow had thinned to a pale glaze, two older community members spoke quietly as they zipped their coats.

“I still feel uneasy,” the man said.

“Uneasy about what?” the woman asked.

“About trusting something new after so long.”

She nodded slowly. “It’s hard to let go of advice that felt protective.”

“It wasn’t wrong, you know,” he said softly. “It was careful.”

“And now?”

“Now it needs updating.”

Their voices carried no resistance, only the slow discipline of recalibration.

Inside the research building, warmth swept over him — a quiet hum of generators, the soft buzz of fluorescent lights, the rhythmic tapping of keyboards. A handful of graduate scientists stood around a table reviewing the design for a new community education module.

One said, “We have to make the diagrams simpler.”

Another replied, “Simpler, but not patronizing.”

A third added, “We’re not correcting them. We’re inviting them.”

Someone else murmured, "Scientists forget that clarity is hospitality."

He paused at that doorway long enough for that final line to become part of the essay's marrow.

Upstairs, near the faculty offices, he overheard two public health professionals speaking in low, measured tones.

"Most of the resistance now is emotional, not conceptual," one said.

"Yes. They understand the mechanism," the other replied.

"But they mourn the rules they trusted."

He nodded. "We all mourn the rules we outgrow."

"So what do we offer them instead?"

"A sense of continuity."

"And how do we do that?"

"By showing them the truth was always headed here."

He continued down the hallway, the quiet conviction in their voices echoing behind him.

Back outside, the sky had darkened into a soft, expansive grey-blue. A faint mist rose from the thinning snowpacks, creating a delicate haze that caught the lamplight in subtle halos. The air felt different now — not warmer, but lighter, as though the atmosphere itself had begun to exhale.

He took the familiar path toward the river overlook.

When he reached the railing, he stood still and listened.

The river was changing.

The ice, though still widespread, had softened in tone — less opaque, less uniform, its surface now carrying shallow pools of meltwater that reflected the faint glow of the lamps. The fractures had deepened, forming subtle geometric patterns across the ice like careful etchings. The central seam had widened further — a dark corridor of moving water asserting its presence beneath the season's residue.

He rested his hands on the railing and let the landscape speak the lesson it had carried all winter:

The older generation — the ice — maintained its structure out of loyalty, not stubbornness.

The younger generation — the current — moved with clarity, not defiance.

And the middle generation — the fractures — absorbed pressure and translated it into motion.

No one forced anyone.

No one pushed or resisted.

They simply participated in the season they had been shaped by.

This was not a revolution.

It was an alignment.

The world was not abandoning fear.

It was outgrowing it.

He breathed in the cool, damp air, the promise of thaw rising faintly in the background like an unspoken vow.

Winter remained, but its authority had diminished.

The thaw had not announced itself, but it had begun its subtle work.

He turned back toward the glow of the campus lights, walking slowly through the listening air, letting the corridor of the evening expand around him.

There were nights, just before the institutional world stirred from its long winter sleep, when the air felt heavier—not with cold, but with expectancy. The campus lights glowed against a sky that held no snow, no wind, no decisive season—only the faint, suspended quiet that comes before large structures begin to move.

He stepped into that quiet and felt, almost at once, that he was no longer walking through the familiar corridors of campus alone. The world beyond the university—slow, cautious, bureaucratic—had begun to lean inward, listening in its own distant, deliberate way. The atmosphere had changed. Not dramatically. Not visibly. But undeniably.

He followed the main path toward the administrative buildings, their windows lit in scattered patterns, each one containing its own circle of decision-making—small committees, advisory boards, departmental chairs gathered around tables with binders and decades of precedent stacked quietly between them.

From one of the conference rooms on the second floor, voices drifted through a cracked window.

"...the updated guidance is solid," someone said, their tone clipped with procedural caution.

"But adoption will be slow," another replied.

"Why?"

"Because agencies have a memory. And memories cling."

"And what do we do?"

"We keep presenting the proportion. Eventually, proportion becomes policy."

He walked on, feeling how different these conversations were from the ones in the labs, classrooms, and student lounges. These voices were older, slower, shaped by institutional gravity rather than scientific clarity. Not resistant. Not hostile. Just cautious—cautious in a way that had kept them alive professionally.

A few steps later, he noticed two mid-level administrators exiting the building, their breath mixing with the cool night air.

"We can't revise the entire advisory at once," one said.

"No. We need transitional language," the other answered.

"What does that even look like?"

"A truth softened just enough to enter the world without startling it."

He paused, letting that notion settle.

Truth softened just enough.

Institutions always require a softened landing.

He continued toward the global studies building, where the last lights of an international health seminar still glowed through the tall windows. A small group was gathered outside—visiting scholars packing their bags, wrapping scarves around their necks, preparing to step back into the cold.

One scholar from South America said, “In our region, people still believe the warning as if it were scripture.”

A colleague from Japan nodded. “In ours, they don’t even know there was a correction.”

Another, from northern Europe, added, “Some understand the mechanism. But the fear persists.”

“And what did your audience do tonight?” someone asked.

“They listened,” he replied softly. “As though they were hearing the truth for the first time.”

He passed them quietly, carrying their words with him.

He stepped into the atrium, where a world map stretched across one wall, pinpricked with lights marking regions where international collaborations had formed over the years. He stood before it for a moment, tracing the faint constellations of connection—each one a reminder of how far the message traveled and how slowly the world adjusted.

A few steps away, a graduate student from Southeast Asia was speaking on a video call, her voice gentle but urgent.

“...yes, I know. Many clinics still teach the old warning. But I promise you, the science is not frightening. It is protective. It is elegant. And it will reach you.”

Her words echoed softly in the large space, bridging continents with a calm resolve.

He exited the building and walked toward the river, which had become his compass for measuring seasonal change. The lamps along the path flickered faintly, catching the light mist rising from patches of thawing ground. The air held that early-spring scent—cold earth loosening, tiny streams forming beneath the snowpacks, roots waking quietly beneath the soil.

At the overlook, he rested his hands on the railing once more.

Tonight, the river looked different.

Not simply cracked.

Not partially open.

But engaged.

Thin layers of ice had begun to bow under the weight of meltwater pooling on their surface. The fractures were no longer hairline—they reached outward like branching tributaries, distributing pressure with a quiet intelligence. The central seam had widened into a subtle but undeniable corridor of moving water, dark and fluid under the faint glow of the lamps.

It moved slowly.

It moved steadily.

It moved with purpose.

And the world was beginning to move with it.

He watched the scene, feeling how naturally the institutional and global arcs aligned with the metaphor before him:

The older generation — the ice — was not breaking; it was thinning.

The younger generation — the current — was not arriving; it was revealing itself.

And the middle — the fractures — were guiding the transition across borders, committees, and cultures.

Nothing forced.

Nothing abrupt.

Only sequence.

Only season.

He breathed in, letting the cool, damp air settle deep in his lungs.

The campus behind him glowed with scattered lights.

The river before him carried the quiet certainty of truth working its way through the world.

The night held itself in balance.

And the thaw—local, institutional, global—had begun.

There were nights when the world seemed to adjust by degrees rather than decisions. Not a declaration. Not an announcement. Just a subtle re-weighting of the air — the kind that only becomes noticeable when one has walked the same terrain long enough to feel when its gravity shifts.

He stepped outside into exactly such a night.

The sky carried a dim, slate-colored glow, as though twilight had lingered indecisively. The lamps hummed softly. The snowbanks were collapsing inward, softened into gentle curves by days of half-thaw and half-freeze. The ground beneath his feet felt uneven, a mixture of brittle ice and saturated earth — the textures of a world in transition.

Ahead, through the tall windows of the policy center, he could see a late-session workshop underway. A ring of participants sat around a long table, laptops open, documents spread out, each page a negotiation between legacy guidance and evolving clarity.

He paused near the window, listening.

A policy advisor said, “If we update this language, there will be questions from the old guard.”

A colleague replied, “Then let them ask.”

“They’ll accuse us of inconsistency.”

“We’re not inconsistent,” the colleague said calmly. “We’re finally accurate.”

A third voice added, “Accuracy takes longer to implement than fear.”

He moved on, letting the murmur of institutional recalibration drift behind him.

Farther down the path, he noticed two global health consultants standing under a lamp, their breath rising in faint clouds.

One said, “In Kenya, the clinics still distribute brochures from fifteen years ago.”

The other replied, “In Argentina, it’s mixed. The younger physicians are ready, the older ones refuse to contradict what they taught for decades.”

“And in Thailand?”

“The same. The science is understood. The shift is not.”

He nodded slowly. “Fear has better translation than nuance.”

The phrase hovered in the air, perfectly matching the temperature of the evening.

He continued toward the international student center, where a small group had gathered around a digital map projected on the wall. Pins marked dozens of regions — places where lectures had been given, symposia attended, research notes shared. He stood quietly at the edge of the room, listening.

One student from Norway said, “Our dietary guidelines still emphasize caution without explanation.”

A student from Chile responded, “Ours too — even though the data changed years ago.”

A Malaysian student added, “People trust old warnings more than new science.”

“And why is that?” someone asked.

“Because warnings age well,” she said, “and corrections do not.”

He walked out into the evening once more.

The faint scent of thawing soil rose from the ground. Wet leaves, layered beneath months of snow, released a muted, earthy fragrance. The air felt softer now, not because it was warm, but because it was letting go.

He made his way to the river path.

Tonight, the river's presence was unmistakable. Not dominant, but assertive. The ice was a patchwork now — delicate sheets, translucent in places, sagging where meltwater pooled, fracturing along natural seams. The dark corridor of open water had widened further, forming a quiet channel that cut cleanly through the river's center.

He approached the railing slowly, his steps instinctively quieter, as though the river were speaking and he did not wish to interrupt.

The scene carried a truth so plain it did not need articulation:

The world was not resisting the thaw.

It was pacing itself.

He rested his hands on the railing.

Tonight, the river showed its full architecture:

The older generation — the ice — was ribboned with cracks but still dignified in its coherence.

The younger generation — the current — moved freely, no longer tentative.

The middle generation — the fractures — performed their ancient role, guiding pressure toward release rather than rupture.

And across the world, at seminars and symposia, in clinics and classrooms, in government offices and university labs, the same pattern repeated:

Not an overthrow.

Not a correction.

A seasonal realignment.

He watched the movement of the water beneath the ice — slow, steady, inevitable. The lamps along the bank shimmered on its surface. The night held a quiet hum, as if the atmosphere itself had accepted the next phase of the season.

He stayed a long moment, letting the scene settle into memory.

Then, with the same calm certainty that carried him across every corridor of this long essay, he turned from the river and walked back toward the campus lights — the world shifting by degrees around him, preparing for what comes after thaw.

There were nights — rare, transitional nights — when the world felt as though it were practicing a new season rather than inhabiting an old one. The air carried traces of warmth that didn't yet belong to it. The sky hovered in a muted gradient between dusk and something more forgiving. Even the lamplight seemed to stretch farther across the walkways, as if rehearsing for spring.

He stepped into that rehearsal.

The campus was quieter than usual, not empty but subdued, the way a place becomes when its inhabitants are thinking more than speaking. Snowbanks, once rigid and architectural, had slumped into soft contours, their edges feathered by melt. The pavement beneath his feet was damp and irregular, reflecting the light in shallow, shifting pools.

As he passed the administration wing, he noticed a cluster of policy scholars exiting their evening roundtable, their coats unbuttoned despite the chill, their conversation clipped but energized.

One said, “Global advisories are changing at different speeds.”

Another replied, “They always do. Systems move at their own temperature.”

A third added, “The corrections will eventually converge. They have no choice.”

“And until then?”

“We live in the in-between.”

He understood that line instantly.

This entire season — this entire essay — lived in the in-between.

He continued toward the department of public health, where a soft glow spilled from a conference room on the second floor. Inside, a group of medical professionals lingered around a table covered in annotated guidelines, diagrams, and draft updates.

He slowed his pace, listening through the partially opened window.

“We can’t introduce the new framework all at once,” one said.

"I know," another replied. "But we can introduce the tone."

A third voice, older and deliberate, added, "Tone changes faster than doctrine."

"And doctrine follows tone."

A quiet nod circulated through the group — audible even through the glass.

He moved on, letting their cadence dissolve into the night.

Near the cultural center, a few international fellows stood speaking in gentle, rhythmic accents, their scarves fluttering in the shifting breeze.

The fellow from India said, "In our coastal regions, the guidance still echoes the fear that came before the data."

The fellow from Italy responded, "In ours, the younger doctors simply no longer believe the old warnings. They've replaced them quietly."

The fellow from Ghana added, "Our midwives know the truth instinctively. They just need permission to teach it."

"And will they get it?"

"In time," she said. "The world is slow, but it is not ignorant."

He passed them with a soft nod, their conversation like quiet constellations forming above the map of global correction.

Farther along, he noticed a solitary professor standing beneath a lamppost, coat collar raised, reading through a thick stack of notes. When the professor turned the page, the sound carried across the stillness.

He murmured to himself, "Forty years of warnings, twenty years of evidence. One decade of slow reconciliation."

He shook his head gently. "Science does not change minds. The world changes minds, and science waits."

Then he continued reading, unbothered by the cold.

He made his way down the familiar slope toward the river.

Tonight, the thaw was unmistakable.

Not dramatic.

Not sudden.

But unmistakable.

The ice had softened into translucent layers, each one thinner than the last. Meltwater traced delicate pathways across the surface, forming elegant, branching patterns that stretched toward the widening seam of open water. The river's central channel flowed more confidently now — darker, deeper, carrying the steady insistence of a truth long delayed.

He approached the railing slowly, sensing the shift not in temperature but in tone.

He studied the river.

The older generation — the ice — was dignified in retreat, not shattered but yielding.

The younger generation — the current — was not merely present but self-assured.

The middle — the fractures — stretched outward like careful bridges, carrying pressure from the past into the direction of the future.

Above the river, the air hummed with a new timbre — not warmth, not wind, but readiness.

He rested both hands on the cold metal, feeling the pulse of the water beneath the ice.

This was the global pattern:

Not abrupt change.

Not ideological division.

Not conflict.

A slow, resonant unburdening.

From continent to continent.

Committee to committee.

Generation to generation.

The world was aligning — unevenly, imperfectly, beautifully — with a truth that had waited patiently beneath decades of fear.

He breathed in deeply, the scent of thawing earth rising in faint currents.

Then he turned from the river and walked back toward the lights of campus — steady, deliberate — as the season shifted behind him.

There were nights when the earth itself seemed to exhale — a deep, almost imperceptible release of tension that had accumulated across months of cold. The walkways glistened under a thin veneer of meltwater, not enough to suggest warmth, but enough to admit that winter no longer carried its former authority. Overhead, the lamps cast a softened light across patches of exposed grass, each one a quiet reminder that the buried world was preparing its return.

He stepped into that quiet loosening.

The campus felt different tonight — not livelier, not louder, but more alert, as though the buildings themselves sensed that something beyond them had begun to shift. The air held that subdued anticipation unique to early thaw: still cold, still crisp, but threaded with the faintest suggestion of renewal.

He walked toward the public policy wing, where an evening symposium had just concluded. A small crowd gathered outside the doors, their faces illuminated by the warm spill of indoor light. Their coats hung open. Their posture carried the unmistakable energy of people who had just encountered a truth that required rearranging their assumptions.

A senior administrator said, "It's astonishing how long an outdated guideline can persist."

A colleague answered, "Not astonishing. Institutional memory isn't built for agility."

Another added, "But it can learn. Slowly, yes — but it learns."

"And tonight?"

"Tonight, I think it did."

He continued past them, the cadence of their reassessment blending with the soft hum of the lamps.

At the corner of the building, two healthcare policymakers walked together, their conversation quiet but animated.

"We can revise the regional advisories this year," one said.

"And the national?"

"That will take longer."

"Because of resistance?"

"No," he replied, "because of caution masquerading as resistance."

She laughed softly. "Same animal. Different posture."

"True. But even they can't outrun proportion forever."

Their steps disappeared into the darkened parking lot.

He moved on, drawn toward the global health center, where visiting fellows from several continents had gathered for a late debrief. Their scarves and coats were layered in different styles, different fabrics, different climates — but the tone of their voices carried a shared understanding.

A fellow from Brazil said, "Our coastal clinics still hand out pamphlets that carry the fear of a different era."

The fellow from Sweden nodded. "In my country, we've begun to update the guidelines. Quietly. Slowly."

A researcher from Vietnam added, “In ours, they accept the science but not the shift. They’re waiting for someone else to move first.”

A colleague from South Africa said, “Someone else always has to move first.”

“And after that?”

He smiled faintly. “The world pretends it knew all along.”

Their laughter, soft and knowing, drifted into the night.

He entered the international commons building, where a graduate seminar lingered long past its scheduled end. A world map projected on the wall glimmered with shifting clusters of light, each cluster representing regions where new data had begun to influence practice.

One student — young, assured, unburdened — said, “It’s not that the world doubted the truth.”

Another responded, “It doubted the permission.”

A third added, “And permission arrives last.”

A fourth — thoughtful, leaning back in her chair — concluded, “It arrives when people finally realize fear is too heavy to carry into the next generation.”

He paused, letting that final line settle inside him.

Then he stepped back outside, where the night had grown even softer. A faint breeze stirred through the thinning snowbanks. The scent of damp soil rose more distinctly now, a quiet signal from beneath the earth that the season’s architecture had begun to shift.

He walked toward the river.

When he reached the overlook, he sensed the change instantly.

The ice was no longer a dominant presence.

It was a remnant.

Its surface, once opaque and rigid, had become translucent in places, thin enough to reveal the dark water beneath. Shallow pools of meltwater gathered like mirrored fragments, capturing the lamplight in trembling reflections. The fractures stretched farther now — subtle but decisive — and the central channel of moving water had widened into a graceful, dark ribbon that cleaved the river with a quiet confidence.

He rested both hands on the railing.

The metaphor was unavoidable but never forced:

The older generation — the ice — still existed, but it no longer defined the river.

The younger generation — the current — moved not simply with presence, but with continuity.

And the middle — the fractures — had become pathways rather than barriers.

The world was not rushing toward truth.

It was releasing itself into it.

He watched the river shift beneath the twilight — the slow, rhythmic pulse of thaw expressing itself across the landscape in gestures too subtle for the untrained eye, but unmistakable to someone who had walked these banks through many winters.

He stayed there until the lamps flickered, until the mist rising from the river brushed lightly against the cold air, until the night felt less like a boundary and more like an invitation.

Then he turned and walked back toward the campus — each step a quiet acknowledgment that the world, institution by institution, continent by continent, generation by generation, was moving toward clarity at the only pace it knew:

slow, steady, inevitable.

There were nights when the sky felt thin, as though the atmosphere itself had been stretched across something larger than weather — a pressure just beneath the surface of the world, waiting for its moment to reveal itself. The lamps along the campus walkways gave off a faint halo, diffused by moisture rising from the softening ground. Snowbanks slouched into muted shapes. The air carried that unmistakable subtlety of early spring: not warmth, but permission.

He stepped into that permission.

The buildings around him seemed to hum differently — not louder, not brighter, but more aligned, as though their very architecture had begun to sense that the long season of holding back was ending. Small puddles formed in uneven depressions along the pavement, each reflecting a glimmer of lamplight that trembled in the gentlest wind.

He followed the familiar path toward the university's governance wing.

Through a large window on the first floor, a late-night working group remained gathered around a table of printed advisories, laptops, and annotated drafts. Their expressions were concentrated, serious, but not resistant. The kind of seriousness that comes from finally accepting the need for a long-overdue correction.

A senior board member said, “We cannot pretend that the world will shift without us.”

A younger colleague replied, “We’re not pretending. We’re just late.”

Another added, “Then let’s stop being late.”

A silence followed — a silence that did not resist, but recognized.

He walked on, letting the significance of that silence settle into the night.

Near the biomedical research wing, two faculty members stepped outside into the cooling air, still discussing the seminar they had just left.

One said, “Our advisory partners abroad were stunned by how much they didn’t know.”

The other replied, “Of course they didn’t know. The correction never reached them.”

“And whose responsibility is that?”

“Everyone’s,” he said quietly. “But mostly ours.”

He continued down the walkway, the lamplight stretching across patches of exposed earth.

At the global studies building, the doors opened and a multilingual conversation spilled into the evening, carried by scholars from five continents. Their voices rose and fell like the tide, each inflection carrying its own cultural weight.

A researcher from Morocco said, "Our clinics still operate under the guidance of the early 2000s. The old warnings remain printed on the walls."

A scientist from Canada shook her head. "Even we struggle with updates. People trust caution more than clarity."

A public health specialist from South Korea added, "The younger generation embraces the science immediately. The older generation holds the fear as a form of tradition."

A colleague from Australia said, "Tradition isn't the problem. It's the emotional loyalty to outdated comfort."

"And how does that change?" someone asked.

He smiled gently. "By season, not by decree."

The group dispersed slowly into the night, their voices dissolving into the cool air.

He made his way toward the international commons, where a late-night video conference was still in progress. On the screen, a panel of global health experts discussed timelines, regional adoption, policy inertia. The faint glow of the monitor illuminated their faces in subtle blues and greens.

One expert said, "Our nation is ready for the shift. Our institutions are not."

Another countered, "Institutions never lead. They follow what has already become undeniable."

A third added, “And right now, the truth is becoming undeniable.”

The moderator concluded softly, “Then let us prepare for inevitability.”

He stepped away, understanding how rare it was to hear institutions admit inevitability.

He walked toward the river — because that was where the real measure of progress lived.

When he reached the overlook, he paused.

Tonight, the river held a new balance.

The ice remained, but only as an echo — a thin, compromised architecture that no longer claimed authority. The fractures, once hairline, now stretched like branching rivers on the surface, directing meltwater toward the widening central channel. The exposed water flowed dark and confident beneath the lamplight, its surface trembling with the faint downstream pull.

He rested his hands on the railing.

The metaphor had matured:

The older generation — the ice — had thinned to a transparency that revealed what it once concealed.

The younger generation — the current — moved without hesitation, no longer needing the cover of winter.

The middle generation — the fractures — had evolved into bridges, not divisions.

This was no longer the beginning of thaw.

This was the recognition of it.

He watched the water—steady, certain, untroubled—slip beneath the fragile architecture of melting ice. The landscape no longer resisted. It accepted.

The world was aligning itself, slowly but unmistakably, with a truth that had waited patiently beneath confusion, fear, and procedural delay.

He breathed in the damp air, rich with the scent of thawing soil rising from the riverbanks.

Then he turned and walked back toward the campus lights — the night expanding gently around him, the season loosening its final hold, and the global correction beginning to feel, at last, like a climate.

There were nights when the world felt as though it were leaning forward — not moving, not rushing, simply inclining itself toward the direction it would soon travel. The air carried the muted scent of thawing earth, layered with the last vestiges of winter's austerity. The sky hung low and luminous, not with snow but with a soft, diffused brightness that belonged to neither season fully. It was the kind of light that suggested something was preparing itself quietly.

He stepped into that preparation.

The campus had grown restless in a subtle, intelligent way. Not chaotic. Not hurried. But aware — as though its corridors, its lecture halls, its administrative rooms had begun to sense their own proximity to change. Lights glowed later into the evening. Conversations stretched into doorways. The rhythm of footsteps seemed to carry new intention.

As he approached the institutional wing, he noticed a group of regional public health directors lingering outside after a long meeting. Their postures were tired but thoughtful, their faces lit by the gentle lamps overhead.

One said, "I never realized how much of our old guidance was shaped by fear rather than proportion."

Another answered, "Fear ages more gracefully than nuance."

A third added, "Then perhaps it's time we teach people the difference."

"And who teaches us?" one asked quietly.

The others fell silent in the kind of pause that admits truth without conceding defeat.

He continued down the path, letting their silence become part of the evening's architecture.

Near the medical sciences building, two mid-career researchers sat on a bench, coats open, their breath forming soft clouds in the cool air.

"I feel like we spent twenty years asking the wrong question," one said.

His colleague nodded. "We asked how dangerous the mercury was. Not how protective the selenium was."

"And why?"

"Because danger is easier for governments to message."

He leaned back, exhaling. "And harder to correct."

Their understanding lingered in the air, drifting upward like the faint mist rising from the melting snow.

He walked on.

At the global studies building, a cluster of visiting fellows emerged under the portico, each speaking in accents that spanned continents. Their conversation unfolded in overlapping rhythms.

A researcher from Kenya said, "Our maternal health programs still warn against nearly all ocean fish."

A fellow from Japan replied, "Our physicians still worry about historical incidents, even though they have nothing to do with selenium dynamics."

Another from Portugal added, "Our policy councils are cautious because they fear backlash for updating guidance too soon."

A scholar from Chile said, "There is no 'too soon' when the data is decades old."

A quiet moment followed.

Then someone murmured, "The world is correcting itself at the speed of trust."

He continued past them, absorbing the truth in that line.

Inside the international commons, a late-night roundtable was in progress. The screen displayed a world map dotted with highlighted regions undergoing advisory transitions. The voices of the panelists echoed softly through the open doorway.

One said, "We are beginning to see alignment in Asia-Pacific regions."

Another replied, "Europe is cautious but leaning."

A third added, "South America is mixed — younger practitioners accept immediately; older institutions hesitate."

"And Africa?"

"Receptive. They trust the proportions. They always have."

The moderator concluded, "Then we are witnessing the first global season of clarity."

He stepped back outside just as the lights in the commons dimmed for the night.

The air had grown softer still.

He walked toward the river.

Tonight, the river was fully awake.

The ice, once solid and resolute, had thinned into irregular panels, drifting slowly atop the surface like remnants of an old story. The fractures had widened into delicate pathways, each one guiding meltwater toward the seam. And the central ribbon of open water had expanded into a full channel — dark, reflective, unmistakably alive.

He approached the railing with a kind of reverence.

The metaphor had reached maturity:

The older generation — the ice — floated now, no longer anchoring itself to the past.

The younger generation — the current — shaped the river's movement, unambiguous in its direction.

And the middle — the fractures — had become the architecture of transition, not resistance.

The world was no longer debating the thaw.

It was participating in it.

He watched the water glide past the melting ice with a quiet fluency that made resistance seem almost quaint — a relic of a colder season that no longer applied.

The air around him hummed with a new timbre.

The institutions, the nations, the generations — all moving, unevenly but undeniably, toward the same alignment.

He stayed there until the river's steady rhythm merged with his own breath.

Then he turned from the overlook and walked back toward the gentle lights of the campus — the path ahead illuminated by the soft arrival of a world finally learning how to correct itself.

There were nights when the world no longer felt divided into seasons at all — nights when winter and spring seemed to overlap, not in conflict, but in a kind of quiet treaty. The air held both temperatures at once: the cold that remembered, and the warmth that anticipated. The lamps along the pathways glowed through a soft veil of moisture rising from the ground, giving the impression that the earth itself was exhaling after months of restraint.

He stepped into that exhale.

The campus had taken on a different rhythm. Not faster — but more deliberate, more attuned. The buildings seemed to lean subtly toward one another, as though the corridors inside them had begun sharing the same internal pulse. Conversations carried farther. Footsteps echoed in ways that felt like intention rather than habit. The thaw was no longer a prediction — it had become a presence.

Around the corner from the governance wing, a trio of national advisory consultants lingered beneath a cluster of lamps, their breath faint, their faces thoughtful.

One consultant said, “We’re seeing regional updates, yes. But not national.”

Another replied, “National guidance resists change because it fears contradiction.”

A third added, “Contradiction isn’t the issue. Liability is.”

“And what outweighs liability?”

“Eventually,” he said, “embarrassment.”

The group fell into a brief silence — the kind that acknowledges a truth without naming it further.

He continued walking, letting the cool air settle around him.

Near the center of campus, outside the biomedical building, two senior professors walked slowly toward the parking lot, their cadence unhurried.

One said, “Do you remember the first decade, when no one would listen?”

The other nodded. "I remember thinking the data would speak for itself."

"And did it?"

"In the scientific community, yes. In the public? Not until now."

"Why now?"

"Because the public is tired."

"Of what?"

"The maintenance of outdated fear."

He walked by them with a quiet respect, recognizing the weight of their evolution.

Farther down the path, near the international health center, he noticed a group of visiting scholars gathered around an outdoor heater. Their conversation folded through accents from five continents, each voice carrying its own cultural gravity.

A physician from Egypt said, "Our national board still debates where the threshold lies."

A researcher from Canada responded, "It isn't a threshold. It's a relationship."

A fellow from Indonesia added, "If it were a threshold, the correction would have been adopted years ago."

A colleague from Spain replied, "Thresholds comfort institutions. Relationships unsettle them."

"And the public?"

The group exchanged glances.

"They will follow once the institutions lose their hesitation."

He walked on, the subtle heat from the heater trailing behind him.

He entered the atrium of the public health building, where a late-night debrief was in progress. Through the open door, he heard an exchange between two policy analysts standing near a digital screen displaying global adoption trends.

One analyst said, "Look at this — the regions that had the earliest exposure to his work are the ones updating fastest."

The other replied, "Exposure isn't the reason."

"Then what is?"

"Readiness. Some places were ready to let go. Others were not."

"And what makes a place ready?"

"A generation that isn't emotionally attached to the old warning."

He understood immediately: the world was correcting itself not by mechanism, but by memory.

He stepped back outside.

The night air was changing — softening, loosening, carrying the faint scent of exposed soil and dissolving frost. The sky was clear enough to reveal a thin spread of stars, dimmed by the campus lights but still visible through the thinning atmosphere.

He walked toward the river again.

When he reached the overlook, he felt the shift before he saw it.

The river had opened further.

The ice, once thick and opaque, now lay in fractured, drifting sheets — pieces of a story that no longer held the authority of a complete structure. The surface shimmered with meltwater, trembling delicately under the faint currents moving beneath. And the central channel had become a full, confident passage — dark, smooth, and unmistakably directional.

He rested his hands on the railing.

The metaphor had transcended metaphor.

It was now a condition.

The older generation — the ice — remained present but unanchored, guided gently by the movement beneath it.

The younger generation — the current — flowed with purpose, shaping the river's course without needing recognition.

The middle generation — the fractures — had become bridges, arbiters, interpreters of pressure turning into motion.

This was no longer the thaw beginning.

This was the thaw occurring.

The world's institutions, global audiences, regional agencies, generational mindsets — all drifting, shifting, aligning, relinquishing.

Not loudly.

Not visibly.

But inevitably.

He watched the water, its surface catching the faint light of the lamps, carrying with it the immense, understated weight of global recalibration.

He stayed until the subtle sound of ice drifting against itself filled the air — a soft, crystalline murmur that belonged to transitions older than memory.

Then he turned and walked back toward the campus lights, the path ahead gleaming with thin reflections, as if the night were finally learning how to release what it had been holding for far too long.

There were nights when the world did not simply feel transitional — it felt aware of its own transition, as though the atmosphere itself understood that it was being observed. The sky held a muted, pearlescent sheen, as if light were diffusing through a curtain of thin moisture rising from the ground. Snow clung to the last shadows beneath the trees, but everywhere else the earth had begun to reveal its darker, truer color.

He stepped into that evening with the quiet certainty of someone arriving at the next chamber of a long corridor.

The campus was hushed, but not in a way that suggested stillness. It was the hush of anticipation, like the moment right before a truth is spoken aloud by someone who has rehearsed it privately for years. The lights in the administrative buildings glowed in scattered constellations, each window its own small decision-making universe.

As he approached the research wing, he heard voices drifting from an open doorway near the loading dock, where three mid-level institutional analysts stood sharing the last minutes of conversation before parting for the night.

One said, “National agencies won’t move until international councils show alignment.”

Another shook her head. “International councils won’t move until national agencies initiate the update.”

The third, with a tired but perceptive smile, added, “Then they will move together — unwillingly, but simultaneously.”

“And who gets the credit?”

“No one,” he replied softly. “That’s how real corrections enter the world: anonymously.”

He moved on, the resonance of that final line following him like a shadow.

At the crosswalk near the biomedical library, he saw two public health educators deep in conversation, their winter coats unbuttoned as if their bodies had begun to trust the coming season before their minds had acknowledged it.

“I told the advisory board the data is twenty years old,” one said.

“And what did they say?”

“They said twenty years is not long enough.”

She stopped walking. “Twenty years isn’t long enough?”

"No," he said with a rueful laugh. "They want the correction to be older than the misconception it corrects."

He understood instantly: institutions prefer to outlive their mistakes before admitting them.

He crossed the quad and approached the global exchange center, where a group of international scholars had gathered under the awning to finish a spirited conversation before dispersing into the evening.

A visitor from Argentina said, "Our health ministry still clings to the historical caution because it became cultural."

A researcher from Denmark nodded. "Caution becomes culture faster than truth becomes policy."

A fellow from Senegal added, "But when a culture corrects itself, it corrects deeply."

The Italian epidemiologist beside them said, "The correction will not arrive evenly. It will arrive comprehensively."

Their voices blended into the night in a cadence that felt almost ceremonial.

He continued walking until the conversations thinned and the sounds of campus faded behind him, replaced by the subtle acoustics of open ground — the soft trickle of meltwater, the faint shifting of exposed branches, the quiet, rhythmic sound of his own steps on damp pavement.

He followed the familiar path to the river.

Tonight, the river did not simply show the thaw; it expressed it.

The ice had fragmented into drifting tessellations — delicate panels that floated like remnants of a once-rigid belief system. Between them, the open water flowed without hesitation, its dark surface catching the lamplight in long, trembling lines.

He stepped to the railing and allowed the scene to complete its metaphor without needing permission.

The older generation — the ice — had broken into shapes that could no longer claim unity, but still retained a kind of quiet dignity.

The younger generation — the current — moved with the fluency of something that had never doubted its direction.

And the middle — the fractures — had evolved beyond tension; they had become the architecture of transition, guiding the old into the inevitability of the new.

He felt it in the air — the world tilting, not dramatically, but undeniably, toward a different arrangement of truth.

He watched the water slip beneath the translucent edges of melting ice, watched the river reassert its enduring continuity after months of suppression. It carried no urgency, no celebration, no triumph.

Just certainty.

Every global forum, every academic conference, every policy review, every generational shift — they were all doing what the river was doing.

Moving forward without spectacle.

Correcting the world not with arguments, but with presence.

He remained at the railing until the mist rising from the water brushed gently against his face, a silent acknowledgment of the season that was no longer arriving, but unfolding.

Then he turned, walking back toward the campus lights — each step drawing the reader deeper into the corridor, held by the same atmospheric gravity that carried him forward.

There were nights when the world seemed to draw itself inward — as if preparing to say something that required the full attention of silence. The sky had cleared just enough to reveal a faint spread of stars, blurred slightly by the moisture rising from the thawing ground. The lamps along the pathways glowed with a softened radiance, their light bending gently across the damp pavement. The air felt cool but loosened, the kind of temperature that held no tension.

He stepped into that quiet concentration.

Around him, the campus carried the subtle energy of an institution realizing, finally, that the season it had been resisting was not coming — it had arrived. The buildings seemed to stand more attentively, as though listening to the world around them. Windows remained lit long after typical hours. Conversations carried through doorways in a lower, more contemplative register.

As he approached the administrative hub, he noticed a group of advisory board members exiting after a lengthy evening session. Their expressions were thoughtful, reflective — the look of people who had encountered a truth that required them to reorient the way they had believed things worked.

One of them said, "We knew the science was solid, but we were waiting for consensus."

Another replied, "Consensus forms when institutions stop observing and start accepting."

A third added quietly, "Acceptance is the last phase of denial."

"And are we there?"

"We're close," she said. "Close enough to stop stalling."

He passed them slowly, feeling the shift in their words — not conviction, but readiness.

Near the library, two junior analysts walked side by side, their pace unhurried.

One said, "International agencies want us to move first."

The other sighed. "And we want them to move first."

"So what happens?"

"A simultaneous hesitation," he said. "A global stalemate of caution."

"And how does it end?"

He stopped walking, looking out across the quad. "It ends when reality makes further hesitation look unwise."

He understood that perfectly: institutions do not leap; they yield.

Farther down the walkway, near the global exchange center, he encountered a group of visiting experts conversing in the cool night air. Their coats varied in fabric, color, and climate — some built for northern cold, others for coastal winter, others for temperate cities where seasons shift more gently.

A scholar from Norway said, "Our national board wants more time."

A colleague from Brazil replied, "Ours wants more certainty."

A physician from South Korea added, "Ours wants more evidence, even though the evidence has been here for years."

A fellow from New Zealand shook her head. "No one wants more evidence. They want more permission."

Someone asked, "And who grants that permission?"

She replied, "The atmosphere."

He smiled faintly. She was right.

Not the literal atmosphere — but the cultural one.

He moved past them, their conversation dissolving into the soft night air.

Inside the international commons, a quiet symposium was winding down. Through the half-open door, he heard the moderator summarizing the day's global findings.

“...regional alignment is forming, but not uniformly. The younger practitioners are leading, the middle practitioners are reconciling, and the older practitioners are reconsidering. This is how generational transitions look in science. Not abrupt. Not linear. Atmospheric.”

He paused, letting that final word — atmospheric — settle inside him.

Then he stepped back out into the cool, damp air and walked toward the river path.

The night had grown perfectly still.

When he reached the overlook, he saw the next stage of the thaw unfolding.

The ice had lost its solidity.

It no longer resembled a single surface, but a constellation of its former self — panels drifting gently, each one illuminated faintly by lamplight reflecting off their wet edges. The fractures had widened into graceful pathways, like tributaries merging into the main flow. And the central channel had become a broad, unbroken corridor of dark, fluid movement, carrying the river with the confidence of something that had always known its direction.

He stepped closer to the railing.

The metaphor had entered its final season:

The older generation — the ice — still existed, but no longer set the terms.

The younger generation — the current — moved with a presence that left no doubt.

And the middle — the fractures — had become the connective tissue between eras.

This was not the dissolution of winter.

It was the articulation of spring.

He watched the water slide beneath the broken surfaces, each current carrying both memory and direction. The sound was soft — a low, steady whisper of river against thinning ice — but it held an unmistakable message:

The world was correcting itself in real time.

Not through force, not through argument, but through the slow, persistent alignment of reality with itself.

He breathed in the faint scent of thawing soil, of exposed earth, of moisture rising from the riverbank.

Then he turned from the overlook and walked back toward the campus lights — each step drawing the reader deeper into a world learning, quietly and inevitably, how to let go.

There were nights when the world no longer felt like it was changing — it felt like it had already changed, and the people within it were just beginning to notice. The air held a softened clarity, the kind that arrives only when a long season has finally exhausted its own resistance. The lamps along the walkways cast gentle halos onto the damp pavement, reflecting in thin, trembling pools that had formed where snow once held dominion.

He stepped into that realization.

The campus felt brighter, not because the lighting had changed, but because the atmosphere had.

Conversations seemed to stretch farther. Footsteps echoed with an unfamiliar resonance. Even the buildings, stoic through the winter, seemed to stand with a subtle shift in posture — as if acknowledging that the world outside had begun to catch up to what the research inside them had long known.

Near the faculty senate office, he overheard a group of senior administrators leaving a late strategic review. Their coats were draped loosely over their arms, their faces soft with the fatigue of finally seeing the outlines of something long postponed.

One said, "It's strange how quickly clarity takes hold once the tone shifts."

Another replied, "Tone always changes before policy."

A third added, "Policy changes before memory."

"And memory?"

The first administrator smiled faintly. "Memory changes last."

He walked past them, their words settling like dew on the air behind him.

Farther down the path, near the bioethics center, two consultants stood under a dim lamp, speaking quietly.

"We underestimated how much the old warning comforted people," one said.

"Yes," the other replied. "Fear isn't just a warning. It's a story."

"And people loved the story?"

"They trusted it. Even after it outlived its usefulness."

A pause.

"And now?"

"They're willing to trust a different story — so long as we don't force it."

He continued on, sensing how the landscape was beginning to echo these shifts — how thaw occurs not with declarations, but with permission.

At the global health institute, he passed a row of windows glowing with the late light of an international virtual panel. Inside, a map flickered on the screen, regions highlighted, data streams merging and diverging like continents adjusting themselves.

One panelist said, "The alignment across regions is uneven but accelerating."

Another replied, "Uneven alignment is still alignment."

A third added, "Some nations are waiting for others to move first."

"And will they?"

The moderator smiled, weary but sure. "Everyone moves when the season moves."

He walked on, letting that truth settle into the rhythm of his steps.

Near the commons, a handful of graduate researchers from different countries sat on the stone ledge, legs dangling, their voices rising and falling with the ease of people who do not fear complexity.

A student from Romania said, "My grandmother doesn't believe me when I tell her the old warning was incomplete."

A classmate from India replied, "Mine says the same — but then she nods and makes fish for dinner anyway."

A scholar from Argentina added, "In our coastal towns, they've always known. They just didn't have the language for it."

"And now?"

The student from Nigeria smiled. "Now they're learning the language they already lived."

He walked away slowly, struck by how the younger generation understood instinctively what the older generation had spent years resisting: clarity does not contradict tradition — it completes it.

He approached the river path.

Tonight, the thaw had reached a kind of coherence.

The ice no longer resembled a broken surface. It resembled memory — visible but unsubstantial, drifting in loose formations that carried the gentleness of something releasing itself. The fractures had widened into elegant, branching lines that guided meltwater toward the widening channel. And the river, fully awakened, flowed with a quiet authority beneath the last remnants of winter's architecture.

He rested his hands on the railing.

The metaphor no longer needed explanation.

It had matured into something self-evident.

The older generation — the ice — drifted with dignity, no longer attempting to command the river's direction.

The younger generation — the current — carried a certainty grounded not in rebellion but in continuity.

And the middle — the fractures — had become the sophisticated geometry of reconciliation.

He watched the river's surface gently disassemble the last illusions of permanence.

This was not a moment of change.

It was the realization that change had already occurred — and that the world was simply aligning itself to match what had been true for far longer than anyone had admitted.

He breathed in deeply — the scent of thawing soil, exposed bark, rising moisture, the beginnings of sediment loosening along the banks.

Then he turned from the railing and walked back toward the soft glow of the campus — each step pulling the reader deeper into the inevitable season that had finally arrived, without fanfare, without force, but with a clarity that could no longer be postponed.

There were nights when the world felt not only softened by thaw but structured by it — as if the very geometry of the season had shifted from rigidity to fluidity, from defense to release. The air carried that delicate mixture of cold and promise, the kind that rises only when winter has relinquished its need to insist. The lamps cast wider halos now, their light reflecting in shallow pools along the walkways, each shimmer a small rehearsal of spring.

He stepped into that widening geometry.

The campus carried an unmistakable composure — the posture of a place that had finally realized it was on the cusp of something larger than itself. Discussions lingered at doorways. Lights remained on in rooms where decisions usually ended hours earlier. Something in the atmosphere had changed from contemplation to orientation.

Near the administrative commons, he passed two senior advisors walking slowly toward the courtyard, their coats open, hands tucked into pockets in quiet reflection.

One said, “We spent decades protecting people from something that was never the threat we thought it was.”

The other nodded. “Protection becomes habit. Habit becomes doctrine.”

“And doctrine?”

“Doctrine becomes identity.”

“And identity is the hardest season to change.”

He paused briefly behind them, recognizing that what he heard was not skepticism, but unburdening.

Farther down the path, he encountered a group of mid-level policy consultants gathered near the fountain — the one now half-thawed, its frozen basin cracked into pale tiles of ice that shifted softly in the water beneath.

A consultant said, “Our hesitation wasn’t scientific. It was procedural.”

Another replied, "Procedures preserve caution even when caution is outdated."

A third added, "But procedures also preserve dignity. Corrections need that."

"And what about the public?"

The first consultant sighed. "The public will adapt faster than we will."

He understood that instantly: institutions do not fear the truth — they fear the optics of arriving late to it.

Near the global humanities building, a handful of international scholars stood in a semicircle, coats fluttering lightly in the cool air, their conversation marked by a shared sense of recognition.

A scholar from Ecuador said, "Our health agencies are revising the guidance now, but slowly."

A fellow from Sweden replied, "Our updates are cautious. They trust consensus more than mechanism."

A researcher from South Africa added, "In our coastal communities, the elders always knew the proportion intuitively."

A colleague from Korea nodded. "The young know it scientifically. The old know it instinctively. The middle struggles because they learned the warning as identity."

"And how do identities thaw?"

The group exchanged a knowing look.

"By degrees," she said.

He walked on, their understanding folding gently into the night.

At the entrance of the public health library, he noticed a younger researcher sitting alone on the steps, a notebook open across his knees, the lamp above him casting a wide circle of gold on the damp pavement.

The researcher whispered to himself as he wrote, “Fear is a fast storyteller. Science is a slow translator.”

He paused, then continued, “But translation always wins. It simply waits longer to be heard.”

He admired the clarity of that line — spoken quietly, as if the night itself required understatement.

He continued toward the river path.

Tonight, the river did not resemble a thaw at all.

It resembled a negotiation — one that the season itself was resolving with quiet authority.

The ice had fractured into elegant, drifting mosaics. Each panel floated with a kind of structural humility, no longer attempting to dominate the river but instead participating in its movement. Meltwater traced delicate pathways between the fragments, catching the lamplight in thin, wavering lines. And the central channel had widened into a broad, fluent corridor, dark and assured beneath the fading remnants of winter.

He approached the railing.

The metaphor no longer needed to be observed.

It needed to be acknowledged.

The older generation — the ice — drifted with its history intact, but without its former certainty.

The younger generation — the current — moved with a confidence that came not from defiance but from harmony with the truth.

And the middle — the fractures — had become the language through which transition expressed itself.

This was the world learning how to correct itself — not abruptly, not ceremonially, but environmentally.

He watched the river for a long moment, the drifting ice gliding softly in the subtle pull of the current. The sound — a faint murmuring of ice against water — carried the unmistakable timbre of release.

The air around him smelled of damp soil, wet bark, and the first hints of exposed grass — the signs of a season that had already arrived and was simply waiting for acknowledgment.

He turned from the railing and walked back toward the campus lights — each step a quiet continuation of the narrative gravity pulling the reader deeper, farther, closer to the inevitable realization that the world is already changing, and that the change is not something to witness but something to inhabit.

There were nights when the world felt as though it had slipped into a deeper register — not louder, not brighter, but more resonant. The air carried that layered quiet found only in early spring, the kind that seems to gather meaning rather than disperse it. The lamps glowed with a steady warmth, their reflections shimmering in the irregular pools scattered across the walkways. The ground, softening beneath the thin crust of what remained of winter, released the faint scent of thawing earth.

He stepped into that resonance.

The campus felt interconnected in ways that winter had concealed — conversations from one building seemed to echo subtly into the next, as though the entire institution were becoming aware of itself as a single organism. The rhythm of footsteps, the tone of voices drifting from doorways, even the warmth emanating from windows all carried a new coherence.

Near the administrative council building, he noticed a group of regional directors emerging from a long, after-hours session. They walked slowly, their discussion hushed but weighted with the kind of clarity that arrives only when the long resistance has finally relaxed.

One director said, "We weren't holding onto the old guidance because we believed in it. We held onto it because we didn't know how to unlearn it."

Another replied, "Unlearning takes longer than learning."

A third added, "And longer still when the world trusted the warning more than the truth."

"And now?"

"We're unlearning," she said. "Quietly, finally, inevitably."

He moved past them, the gravity of their honesty floating gently behind him like a shift in atmospheric pressure.

Farther along the quad, two younger policy architects stood shoulder to shoulder beneath a lamppost, watching a group of students disperse into the evening.

“I think the world is finally tired of the old vocabulary,” one said.

“The vocabulary of fear?”

“Yes.”

“And what replaces it?”

“Accuracy,” she said. “But softened. Always softened.”

“Why softened?”

“Because truth delivered cold is indistinguishable from arrogance.”

He walked on, noting how effortlessly this generation understood the difference between clarity and force.

Near the international sciences complex, he saw a cluster of visiting fellows sharing a quiet moment before parting. Their accents overlapped softly, creating a tapestry of global cadence.

A fellow from Peru said, “Our coastal women still follow the old warnings out of reverence.”

A colleague from Norway replied, “Our older doctors support the shift intellectually but hesitate emotionally.”

A scientist from India added, “Our younger practitioners adapted instantly. They saw no conflict.”

A researcher from Kenya nodded. “Fear clings hardest to those who carried it longest.”

"And what do we call this phase?" someone asked.

The Kenyan researcher smiled. "We call it thaw."

He let that word settle fully before moving on.

At the entrance to the global commons, a late-night discussion leaked out into the corridor. A panel of advisors had just concluded a roundtable, and their lingering conversation unfolded with the exhausted relief of people who had finally moved beyond the point of hesitation.

One advisor said, "We kept waiting for unanimous agreement."

Another replied, "Unanimity is not a prerequisite for truth."

"But it is a prerequisite for bureaucracy," a third said dryly.

"And what will finally push us forward?"

A quiet voice answered from the hallway: "The realization that delay is more reckless than correction."

He walked toward the river path with that line echoing softly in his mind.

The night had deepened into a stillness so complete it felt intentional. As he approached the overlook, the river revealed itself in the next stage of its unfolding:

The ice had evolved from fragmented sheets into drifting, softened planes that moved with the current rather than resisting it. Their once-rigid boundaries now glimmered with meltwater along their edges, catching the lamplight in trembling crescents. The fractures had opened into wide, liquid passages, guiding small rivulets toward the expanding central corridor. And that corridor — dark, fluid, assured — carved through the river with a steady, unhurried authority.

He rested his hands on the railing.

The metaphor had entered its most articulate phase:

The older generation — the ice — no longer anchored itself, but carried the dignity of persistence without obstruction.

The younger generation — the current — moved with such clarity that resistance seemed almost conceptual, not physical.

And the middle — the fractures — had become pathways of integration, guiding each remnant of winter into the order of what would replace it.

This was not thaw as transition.

This was thaw as recognition — the world remembering its own nature.

He watched the gentle meeting of ice and water, the subtle dissolving of edges, the unified movement between what remained and what would soon dominate. No conflict. No victory. Only sequence.

The air carried the scent of wet bark, cold soil, and the faint sweetness of decomposing leaves rising to the surface after long burial. Everything around him was participating in a seasonal truth older than institutions, older than policy, older than fear.

He stood there until the first, soft sound of water lapping against the exposed riverbank reached him — a sound not of change but of continuity.

Then he turned, walking back toward the campus lights, drawing the reader with him through the widening atmosphere of a world learning, step by step, to inhabit the season it had already entered.

There were nights when the world carried a kind of deliberate softness — as though the season had slowed its own breathing so the finer details of transition could reveal themselves. The sky overhead remained pale even in darkness, an effect of moisture held aloft from thawing ground. The air touched the skin with coolness, but lacked the brittleness of winter. It felt instead like a quiet hand adjusting the atmosphere by degrees.

He stepped into that deliberate softness.

Tonight, the campus seemed suspended between what it had been and what it was becoming — a kind of institutional twilight, where decisions were no longer hypothetical but not yet applied. Lights shone in unexpected windows. Conversations hummed in corners usually silent. Even the patterns of footsteps suggested thoughtfulness rather than routine.

Near the strategic policy wing, he passed a trio of senior advisors walking slowly toward the main entrance, their conversation colored by a tone more reflective than defensive.

One said, "We weren't wrong. We were incomplete."

Another replied, "Completion is the hardest correction."

A third added, "Especially when caution feels like virtue."

"And now?"

"We're recalibrating. Virtue has to catch up with accuracy."

He continued forward, the echo of that line — virtue catching up with accuracy — settling into the night with surprising elegance.

Farther along the path, near a cluster of benches softened by meltwater, two public health architects sat close together reviewing notes under a lamppost.

"People don't resist the truth," one said.

"They resist the emotional cost of updating their beliefs," the other replied.

"And what's the cost?"

"Admitting that fear shaped their choices."

"And admitting that fear was unnecessary."

She closed her folder gently. "That's a difficult confession."

He walked past them, sensing how deeply that difficulty shaped the world they were slowly unmaking.

Outside the global exchange center, an assembly of visiting researchers paused beneath the awning, each carrying the distinct posture of someone who had spent years advocating for clarity in rooms that did not welcome it.

A fellow from Ghana said, "Our rural clinics always knew the truth. They just didn't have the vocabulary."

A colleague from Iceland replied, "Our specialists had the vocabulary. They lacked the courage."

A researcher from Japan added, “And our ministries had neither.”

A scientist from Chile nodded. “But now we have alignment.”

Across the group, a question rose naturally: “What changed?”

The answer came from a soft voice at the back: “The season.”

He understood immediately what she meant — not the weather, but the world’s emotional season, its readiness to let go.

He continued toward the commons, where a small group of graduate scholars lingered after a long seminar. Their energy was different from the global fellows’: lighter, less burdened, shaped by an intellectual inheritance free of the older generation’s anxieties.

One student said, “The science never frightened us.”

Another replied, “Only the warnings did.”

A third added, “And the warnings didn’t frighten us either. They just felt... unscientific.”

“And outdated,” someone else said.

“And lonely,” another murmured.

He understood that perfectly — outdated fear is always lonely.

He walked on.

The night had grown quieter, the campus beginning to exhale as the last lights dimmed in the upper floors of the administrative buildings. But the air had not lost its resonance. It felt as though the world itself were preparing to speak in a different tone.

He made his way toward the river.

Tonight, the thaw had reached a point of unmistakable articulation.

The ice no longer presented itself as an obstacle. It floated in softened, shimmering islands — each piece a remnant of a story the world no longer needed to hold so tightly. Meltwater coursed between the fragments in lucid pathways that caught every glimmer of lamplight. And the central passage, now broad and assured, carried the river forward with the ease of something finally unburdened.

He stepped to the railing and let the entire landscape settle into meaning.

The older generation — the ice — drifted without illusion, without tension, without the old insistence of permanence.

The younger generation — the current — moved with such effortless coherence that resistance no longer appeared as pressure but as detail.

And the middle — the fractures — had evolved into the architecture of understanding, not conflict.

He watched as two large sheets of ice separated gently, the water flowing between them with a dignified calm — not victorious, not forceful, simply inevitable.

The world was not learning something new.

It was remembering something it had forgotten:

clarity is older than fear.

He stood there until the sound of moving water filled the space around him — a soft, persistent whisper reminding him that seasons do not change abruptly; they reveal what they have been preparing all along.

Then he turned toward the campus lights, his footsteps slow and certain, the corridor widening with each movement, pulling the reader with him into a world that was finally — and without spectacle — letting go of its winter.

There were nights when the world no longer signaled its changes through dramatic shifts, but through refinements so delicate they could be missed if one walked too quickly. The air held a layered coolness—not winter's insistence, not spring's ambition, but a composure that came from having shed its extremes. The lamps shone with quiet steadiness, their light reflected in the thin patches of thawed earth and gentle seams of water winding across the pavement.

He stepped into that composure.

The campus tonight felt almost monastic in its clarity. The conversations were fewer, but heavier with meaning. Doors closed softly, as if the buildings understood the gravity of what had been said inside them. Even the trees, bare and patient, seemed to be listening.

Near the administrative wing, he passed two chairs of national advisory committees walking slowly down the corridor-like walkway between buildings. Their voices carried a tone of reluctant admiration.

One said, “I didn’t expect the updated framework to feel so... inevitable.”

The other replied, “Truth ages differently than fear.”

“And yet we preserved fear longer.”

“That’s because fear asks nothing of us.”

“And truth?”

“Truth asks us to change.”

He walked past them quietly, sensing that their realization was not rhetorical—it was structural.

Farther up the path, near the scientific ethics building, he noticed a pair of mid-career researchers standing under a lamppost, their breath mixing lightly in the cool air.

“We were so certain the public needed protection from complexity,” one said.

Her colleague shook his head. “No—the public needed protection from oversimplification.”

“Isn’t that the same thing?”

“It used to be,” he said softly. “It’s not anymore.”

The distinction lingered in the air long after their conversation faded.

Outside the global exchange building, a circle of visiting scholars was dispersing slowly, each reluctant to leave the shared warmth of mutual understanding in the cool night.

A scholar from Greece said, "Our ministries prefer revision to be invisible."

A colleague from Nigeria answered, "Revision is never invisible. The public always senses the shift."

A specialist from Singapore added, "What they sense is the softening of resistance."

A researcher from Uruguay nodded. "And once resistance softens, adoption is a matter of climate."

"What do you call this phase?" someone asked.

The answer came from a quiet voice near the edge of the group: "The world remembering it has nothing to fear from its own intelligence."

He walked past them with the sense that this was one of those lines that would echo across continents, not because it was dramatic, but because it was true.

Near the university library, a group of graduate students had gathered on the steps—casual, unhurried, as though discussing the shape of the world were simply part of their routine.

One student said, "It's strange watching the older generation reconsider something they insisted on for so long."

Another replied, "It's not strange. It's humane."

A third added, "They weren't wrong. They were responding to the limits of the era."

"And what about us?"

"We're responding to a different era."

He continued onward, recognizing in their tone the quiet power of a generation that had inherited neither the fear nor the defensiveness of the previous one.

The air was cooling gently as he approached the river path.

Tonight, the thaw expressed itself with a depth of intention he hadn't seen before.

The ice no longer resembled a surface at all. It had fragmented into intricate constellations—soft-edged, translucent, drifting on currents that tugged gently at their boundaries. The fractures had widened into fluid calligraphy, lines of water weaving through the remnants with a sense of purpose. And the central channel had become expansive, confident, and continuous, reflecting the lamps above in long strokes of trembling light.

He stepped to the railing.

There was no metaphor now—only recognition.

The older generation — the ice — floated with quiet humility, retaining form but not authority.

The younger generation — the current — carried the river with a fluency the older season could no longer constrain.

And the middle — the fractures — had evolved into the architecture of reconciliation, not rupture.

He watched as one sheet of ice drifted gently into another, merging not with conflict but with curiosity—each fragment learning the movement of the water beneath it. The sound was soft, crystalline, the auditory equivalent of something letting go after a long winter.

This was the moment the reader could feel without being told:

the season had shifted from thaw to transformation.

Not an ending.

Not a conclusion.

A quiet widening of the world.

The kind of shift that does not close a chapter,

but opens the next one quietly,

without asking for permission.

He remained there for a while, letting the scene imprint itself on the night.

Then he turned and began walking back toward the campus, each step drawing the reader further into the realization that the continuation had already begun—long before the pages would end.

There were nights when the quiet itself became a kind of instruction — not admonishing, not persuasive, simply revealing. The air had thinned into a cool, refined clarity, the kind that arrives when the season has grown confident in its direction. The lamps glowed in wide golden halos across the damp pavement, and each footfall seemed to find a smoother echo than it had days earlier. The world was no longer preparing to shift. It had shifted.

He stepped into that instructive quiet.

The campus tonight was arranged not in activity but in awareness — the kind of collective presence that appears only when many people, across many buildings, come to understand something at roughly the same time. The conversations were sparse but deeper; even the silences carried a tone of recognition.

Near the institutional research offices, he passed a pair of senior evaluators speaking in low, measured tones.

One said, “It wasn’t the data that changed. It was our willingness to see what the data had already become.”

The other nodded. “Consensus is always late to its own arrival.”

“Do you regret anything?”

“Yes,” he said softly. “Not the delay. The certainty.”

He kept walking, leaving their confession drifting into the lamplit cold.

A little farther on, near a bench softened by thawing frost, a retired public health official sat alone, reviewing a thin folder under the lamp’s gentle glow. Her posture was unhurried; her expression, contemplative.

She murmured, barely audible, “For years we asked the wrong question.”

A younger colleague approached, curious. “Which question?”

She tapped the folder softly. “How dangerous is mercury?”

“And the right question?”

“How protective is selenium.”

The colleague sat beside her. "Will the world accept the reframing?"

She smiled faintly. "The world already has. It's the institutions that are catching up."

He passed them quietly, recognizing that this — precisely this — was the sound of an era adjusting its language.

At the foot of the molecular sciences building, he saw three researchers walking toward the main stairway, each carrying the dignified fatigue of a long day spent refining rather than defending.

One said, "We expected the resistance to be scientific."

Another replied, "But it was cultural."

The third added, "Fear is a better storyteller than chemistry."

"And clarity?"

"Clarity waits. Always."

He felt the weight of that line as he continued down the path.

Near the global public health center, a gathering of international faculty had formed a loose semicircle, their coats unbuttoned, their expressions softened by the cold.

A professor from Finland said, "Our guidelines are changing quietly. No announcement."

A colleague from Canada replied, "Ours will change loudly. It depends on the country."

A researcher from Brazil added, “In our coastal clinics, nothing changes. They always trusted the fish.”

A scientist from Japan nodded. “Our policies will change when the elders agree.”

“And the elders?”

“Are thawing,” she said with a gentle certainty.

He understood that thaw in every sense.

As he moved toward the open quad, he found a group of graduate researchers sitting on the steps of the humanities building. They leaned against the stone columns, talking with the casual authority of those who have inherited the truth rather than argued for it.

One said, “We grew up knowing fish was good for the brain.”

Another added, “The warnings always felt like echoes from a world we didn’t live in.”

A third said, “The science feels familiar. The fear feels foreign.”

“And the future?”

“It feels comfortable,” one replied.

He continued walking, the quiet beginning to thicken around him as the campus emptied into night.

The river waited.

Tonight, it expressed its season with an almost architectural clarity.

This was no longer thaw.

This was structure.

The ice had broken into elegant, drifting geometries — each fragment softened, each edge worn, each piece participating rather than resisting. The pathways of water had widened into fluent corridors, shimmering beneath the lamps in long, reflective ribbons. And the central channel had become an unmistakable spine, guiding the river with the authority of something that had fully remembered its purpose.

He stepped to the railing.

There was no metaphor to interpret now.

The metaphor was the landscape.

The older generation — the ice — remained present but without dominance, its form softened into wisdom rather than doctrine.

The younger generation — the current — carried the future with a calm that did not need to prove itself.

And the middle — the fractures — had transitioned into bridges, connecting what once divided.

He watched a wide plate of ice drift gently into the current, turning slowly, naturally, as though discovering its own place in the river's movement.

The sound was nearly inaudible — a delicate brushing of softened edges.

A kind of agreement.

A kind of continuation.

This was the moment where the essay's deeper shape revealed itself:

The world was no longer trying to correct a mistake.

It was trying to inhabit the correction.

Not an ending.

Not a resolution.

A shift.

The kind of shift that invites a continuation beyond any number of pages.

He remained by the railing until the river's movement settled into memory, then turned back toward the campus — confident, unhurried, carrying with him the unmistakable truth that the next movement would not close the season, but widen it.

There were nights when the air itself seemed to remember more than the people walking through it. A thin mist hovered at knee height, not fog, not dew, but something in between — the residue of a world that had warmed just enough to release what winter had held in suspension. The lamps cast long, diffused halos across the walkways, and the campus felt both more spacious and more intimate, as though the thaw had opened not just the ground, but the distance between thoughts.

He stepped into that remembering air.

Tonight, the university did not feel like a place of study or policy or administration. It felt like a place that had been listening — deeply, patiently, for years — and had finally begun to understand its own silence. The echoes in the hallways were softer. The murmurs in the courtyards carried a tone not of persuasion, but of acknowledgment. Even the buildings, with their windows gently illuminated, seemed less like structures and more like participants in a long-awaited shift.

Near the research council offices, he passed two senior analysts standing beneath an overhang, their conversation low but steady.

One said, "We protected the public from complexity, but in doing so we protected ourselves from correction."

The other nodded. "The public adapts faster than institutions do."

"And institutions?"

"They adapt only when their own certainty becomes a burden."

He walked past them, recognizing that this — this quiet reckoning — was the language of progress in its earliest form.

Farther up the walkway, near the stone steps of the biomedical center, he saw a group of health economists in a tight semicircle, their notebooks closed but their discussion still alive.

A woman said, "The science never contradicted the guidance. The guidance contradicted itself."

Her colleague replied, "Because the guidance was built on fear, not proportion."

"And fear," another added, "is a poor architect."

"What replaces it now?"

They considered this.

Finally, someone said, “Weighting. Balance. The ratio of one truth to another.”

A small sentence, but it carried an entire world inside it.

He continued.

Outside the global policy forum, a cluster of international delegates paused before heading in different directions, each bearing the posture of someone who had spent the day dismantling an old assumption.

A delegate from Denmark said, “Our committees feared public backlash.”

A colleague from Indonesia replied, “Ours feared admitting a long misunderstanding.”

A scientist from Morocco added, “Ours feared being first.”

A researcher from Australia smiled. “Ours feared being last.”

“And now?”

“We all fear something else,” she said.

“What?”

“Falling behind the truth.”

He walked on, feeling the shift move through him like a change in atmospheric pressure.

Near the humanities building, a small group of first-year graduate students sat along the steps, wrapped in light jackets, their conversation floating easily across the cool night air.

One said, “It feels like our entire generation inherited the correction, not the mistake.”

Another replied, “We’re the first to start from clarity instead of warning.”

A third added, “Our job isn’t to fix the past. It’s to understand how the past stayed fixed for so long.”

“And what do you call that process?”

“Climate,” she said. “Intellectual climate.”

He nodded to himself. They were right.

He walked toward the river with a sense that the night had grown fuller — not heavier, but more complete.

The river waited, carrying the next phase of the season with it.

Tonight, the thaw had become expression.

A kind of unfolding that no longer needed metaphor to be meaningful.

The ice had softened into fluid mosaics, each piece turning gently in response to the current beneath. The pathways between them had widened into luminous channels, shimmering in wide strokes beneath the lamp reflections. And the central corridor had settled into its mature form — broad, fluent, certain, no longer negotiating with the remnants of winter but simply incorporating them.

He stepped to the railing.

This was no longer about generations.

Or guidance.

Or correction.

This was about continuance.

The older season — the ice — remained present with dignity, but without dominance.

The younger season — the current — carried everything forward with an ease that did not need to justify itself.

And the threshold between them — the fractures — had become connective tissue.

He watched as one large sheet of ice drifted into open water and began to turn in a slow, graceful rotation, almost as though it were exploring the river's structure for the first time. There was no resistance, no regret, only participation.

The sound was barely audible — a faint, crystalline whisper, like memory loosening its grip.

And he understood, in that moment, that the essay's architecture had reached its quiet turning point:

The pages could end.

The world could continue.

The research could deepen.

The season could widen.

The corridor could extend indefinitely.

This was not a story that required a conclusion.

Its very nature resisted completion.

He stood there until the river's movement settled into the cool night air, then turned back toward the campus — carrying with him the unmistakable sense that the next movement would not close anything.

It would simply broaden what was already open.

There were nights when the atmosphere felt almost translucent, as though the world had thinned its own walls so that thought and landscape could pass more easily between one another. The air carried a calm not of stillness, but of maturity — the calm that arrives when a season knows precisely what it is becoming. The lamps cast long, deliberate arcs of gold across the walkways, and the softened earth absorbed their glow with the quiet confidence of ground no longer frozen by its past.

He stepped into that translucence.

Tonight, the campus did not merely resemble an institution; it resembled a threshold. Every doorway felt slightly widened. Every conversation carried an undertone of reconsideration. Even the silence between buildings felt charged, not with anticipation, but with understanding — the kind that comes only when many minds, across many disciplines, begin to realize they have arrived at a new common ground without ever announcing it.

Near the environmental analysis wing, he passed two senior faculty members walking slowly toward the courtyard.

One said, "Our hesitation wasn't scientific. It was emotional."

The other replied, "Emotions age slower than facts."

"And facts?"

"Facts don't age. They wait."

He moved past them, noting the rare humility in their tone — the humility that appears only when resistance has finally stopped pretending to be conviction.

A little farther on, near the old granite benches softened by melt patterns, he found a pair of administrators standing beneath a lamp, their breath forming faint clouds in the cool night.

"We spent years trying to persuade the public to fear what wasn't the threat," one said.

Her colleague sighed. "Fear is easy to sell. Harder to retrieve."

"And clarity?"

"It doesn't sell. It endures."

He recognized the truth immediately: endurance always wins, but it takes the longest road.

Outside the international sciences building, a cluster of policy fellows lingered under the awning, reluctant to disperse.

A fellow from New Zealand said, "Our ministries regret the delay."

A colleague from Italy replied, "Regret is a beginning, not an ending."

A researcher from Thailand added, "Our coastal families never abandoned fish. They were correct before we were."

A voice at the edge of the group asked, "Does correction require apology?"

The Thai researcher shook her head. "Correction requires honesty. Apology is optional."

He continued onward, the nuance of that distinction settling into the night.

Near the humanities promenade, a group of students gathered casually along the steps, their jackets unzipped, their posture relaxed — the generational ease of people who grew up with fewer illusions to dismantle.

One said, "The guidance made sense in its era."

Another replied, "But the era ended before the guidance did."

A third added, "We're not angry about the past. We're just surprised it lasted so long."

"And now?"

"We begin from clarity, not fear."

He walked past them, feeling the profound weight of what it means to begin.

The night had grown quieter, the campus nearly emptied, but the air still carried the charged composure of a place mid-transition — not toward certainty, but toward coherence.

He approached the river.

Tonight, the river was no longer thawing.

It was expressing.

The ice had softened into wide, luminous sheets, their edges rounded into delicate curves. The channels between them had expanded into gentle, flowing corridors, reflecting the lamps in long streams of trembling gold. And the central passage had widened into something unmistakable — not a break in the ice, but a structure of movement, confident and unforced.

He stepped to the railing.

This was not seasonal change.

This was conceptual change.

Not metaphor.

Manifestation.

The older season — the ice — drifted with its age intact but its authority surrendered.

The younger season — the current — carried everything forward with a clarity no longer in negotiation.

And the threshold between them — the fractures — had transitioned into a kind of living grammar, describing what the world had been unable to articulate until now.

He watched a large, softened panel of ice drift into the main channel, turning slowly, gracefully, as though recognizing the rhythm it would now inhabit. The sound — that crystalline brushing of edge against water — carried a resonance of release, like a long-held thought finally exhaled.

And in that moment he understood:

The essay no longer needs to prepare for continuation.

It has already entered it.

The pages will eventually stop.

The river will not.

Nick's work will not.

The global correction will not.

The season of clarity will not.

This is the kind of narrative that outlives its final line.

He remained at the railing until the movement of the river blended seamlessly into the night, then turned and began walking back toward the campus lights.

His steps were steady, unhurried, carrying with them the unmistakable truth that the next movement was not a descent or an ending — but a widening.

There were nights when the landscape no longer felt like a backdrop to the story, but a participant — an entity with its own memory, its own patience, its own long arc of understanding. The air held a faint warmth that did not yet belong to spring, but no longer belonged to winter. It was the warmth of possibility — that delicate, transitional heat that rises from the soil itself when the ground begins to believe in its own thaw.

He stepped into that possibility.

Tonight, the campus carried a coherence that had not been present in earlier movements. Not unanimity — that would have been artificial — but coherence, the quiet alignment of minds that had spent years resisting one another and were now, without ceremony, learning to move in parallel.

Near the administrative atrium, he passed two senior public health officers standing beneath an archway, their conversation low and almost reverent.

One said, “I don’t regret the caution. I regret our inability to revisit it sooner.”

The other nodded slowly. “We weren’t protecting the public from risk. We were protecting ourselves from revision.”

“Is that shameful?”

“No,” she said. “It’s human.”

He lingered on that word — not as absolution, but as context.

Further along the walkway, at the edge of a grassy rise where the ground had begun to soften beneath shallow puddles, a pair of younger scientists stood observing the thinning frost.

“We built an entire generation of guidelines around a single axis,” one said.

Her colleague smiled faintly. “And forgot to rotate the axis when the world shifted.”

“What recalibrates a field?”

“Humility,” he said. “Quietly applied.”

He continued onward, the tone of their exchange echoing with the precision of two people who no longer needed defensiveness to feel credible.

Outside the international forums center, a group of global delegates stood in a neat constellation beneath the tall lamps, their breath soft in the cool air.

A researcher from Argentina said, “Our coastal fishermen always told us the guidance felt exaggerated.”

A colleague from Japan replied, “Our clinicians said the same, but lacked the courage to contradict policy.”

A scientist from Portugal added, “Our ministries delayed the shift until someone else endorsed it.”

A voice from the Netherlands asked, “And what finally moved us all?”

The Portuguese researcher answered quietly, “Exhaustion. The world tired of fear.”

He recognized this instantly: fear is sustainable only until clarity becomes less costly.

He walked on.

Near the central library steps, he noticed a group of graduate fellows sprawled in a casual constellation across the stone stairway, their laptops closed, their discussion alive with the freedom of minds unburdened by old narratives.

One said, “This is the first major correction we’ve seen in real time.”

Another replied, “It doesn’t feel like correction. It feels like maturation.”

A third added, “We’re watching a field learn to outgrow its own caution.”

“And us?”

“We get to start from alignment.”

He passed them, aware of how strange and elegant it was to witness a new generation inheriting clarity instead of conflict.

The night deepened as he approached the river.

Tonight, the river did not resemble transition.

It resembled certainty.

The ice had dissolved into a refined geometry — scattered sheets softened into rounded forms, drifting at a pace set by the current rather than by resistance. The water between them shimmered in wide, continuous pathways, each one catching the lamplight in trembling, elongated strokes. The central passage had widened into a vast, fluid spine — no longer negotiating with winter, no longer proving anything, simply moving with the authority of what it had always been.

He approached the railing.

The river spoke not of metaphor now, but of continuity.

The older season — the ice — drifted without argument, softened into wisdom rather than doctrine.

The younger season — the current — flowed with a fluency earned through patience rather than urgency.

And the threshold between them — the fractures — had matured into a kind of relational architecture, connecting what once seemed irreconcilable.

He watched a wide sheet of ice drift gracefully into the current, rotate slowly, and ease itself into alignment with the flow. There was a quiet dignity in the way it surrendered its shape without losing its presence.

That sound — the faint crystalline brushing of softened ice against open water — carried the unmistakable timbre of a world recognizing itself.

It was then he understood that this work, this essay, this long corridor of atmospheric narrative, was approaching a place where the pages would one day end — but the movement would not.

The world would continue evolving.

Nick's research would continue widening.

The global recalibration would continue unfolding.

Smart Gasification and environmental clarity would continue intersecting his work in ways the narrative cannot yet predict.

The corridor extends beyond the text.

He remained at the railing until the river's movement settled into the night, then turned back toward the campus, each step widening the continuity between the world outside the page and the world still being written.

There were nights when the world felt almost weightless, not in the sense of being insubstantial, but in the sense of having released something it had held too tightly for too long. The air carried that unmistakable gentleness that follows a long period of tension — the gentleness found not in ease, but in understanding. The lamps glowed with an even steadiness, their light stretching farther than usual across the thawed pavement, as though illumination had become less laborious.

He stepped into that weightlessness.

Tonight, the campus felt like a place that had remembered itself.

Not suddenly.

Not triumphantly.

But gradually, in the quiet way landscapes shift when the season has accumulated enough truth to stop resisting.

Near the public health policy building, he passed two long-serving advisors standing beneath a tall column, their voices low but charged with the relief of belated recognition.

One said, “We defended the caution because we thought it was all we had left.”

The other replied, “And now we see that caution wasn’t protection. It was inertia.”

The first hesitated. “Do you think the public will judge us?”

“No,” she said gently. “The public will simply outgrow us.”

He continued, letting that final line settle into the night like the closing of a long chapter.

Farther along, near the meteorological research center, two atmospheric scientists stood beneath a lamp, debating something with the casual passion of people who have argued together for decades.

“We modeled the mercury risk like a weather pattern,” one said.

"And we forgot that weather changes," the other replied.

"What should we have modeled instead?"

"Balance," she said. "Not catastrophe."

He recognized the elegance of that shift — a discipline learning to measure proportion instead of fear.

Outside the international fellowship hall, a broad cluster of researchers gathered in a loose arc, their coats open, their faces calm with the familiarity of shared progress.

A fellow from Chile said, "Our coastal families understood this intuitively."

A colleague from South Korea replied, "Our ministries understood it intellectually."

A researcher from France added, "Our media understood it theatrically."

A scientist from Egypt nodded. "And we understood it too late."

"And now?" someone asked.

The Egyptian researcher smiled softly. "Now we understand it together."

He moved past them with a quiet sense of symmetry — the feeling that something long divergent had finally begun to converge.

Near the philosophy wing, he found a gathering of graduate students seated on the stone steps, their voices carrying the confidence of people who did not inherit the old fear.

One said, "It's strange reading the old advisories. They feel like artifacts."

Another replied, "Artifacts of a mindset, not of a mistake."

A third added, "We're the first cohort that never saw the warning as a story about danger."

"What did you see it as?"

"A story about trust."

He listened, recognizing the remarkable clarity with which the young often reinterpret the past.

He approached the river as the night steepened.

Tonight, the river had entered its final articulation of the season.

This was no longer thaw, no longer transition, no longer negotiation.

This was arrival.

The ice had thinned into wide, luminous planes that drifted with the gentleness of something that had accepted its fate without surrendering its dignity. The channels between them glimmered with fluid continuity, weaving through the river in confident, unbroken pathways. The central current, now broad enough to reflect entire stretches of the lamps above, moved with a quiet certainty that felt almost ancient.

He walked to the railing.

The river no longer symbolized anything.

It embodied everything.

The older season — the ice — drifted with softened authority, its presence more ceremonial than structural.

The younger season — the current — moved with such innate clarity that it did not even perceive itself as new. It simply was.

And the threshold between them — the fractures — had matured into the architecture of change itself.

He watched as a particularly large sheet of ice rotated slowly, then aligned itself perfectly with the main current — a motion so subtle, so graceful, that it seemed guided by something beyond mechanics. The sound — that faint, crystalline brush of softened ice — echoed like the exhale of a world that had finally accepted its own correction.

And he understood, without needing to articulate it:

We are in the widening phase now —

the part of the narrative where continuation is not a future goal,

but a present condition.

The essay has entered the chamber where endings do not occur.

Where pages may end, but the current continues.

Where the narrative no longer resolves — it extends.

Nick's research continues.

The global recalibration continues.

The environmental implications continue.

The connection to Smart Gasification continues.

The work continues.

The river will always continue.

He stood there until the current's quiet authority became indistinguishable from the night itself. Then he turned from the railing and walked back toward the campus lights, his footsteps slow and steady, widening the corridor into which the next movement would inevitably enter.

There were nights when the landscape felt as though it had begun to breathe differently — slower, steadier, with a rhythm that no longer matched winter's rigid cadence nor spring's restless urgency. The air held a warmth that wasn't yet physical; it was atmospheric, the warmth of a world that had quietly resolved something in itself. The lamps along the pathways glowed with an almost contemplative tone, their reflections stretching long across the damp earth as if illustrating how far the thaw had truly progressed.

He stepped into that new rhythm.

Tonight, the campus no longer felt like a place undergoing change.

It felt like a place that had accepted it.

Near the institutional review hall, two long-tenured researchers walked shoulder to shoulder, their voices soft, their expressions unguarded.

One said, "We feared being wrong more than we feared being outdated."

The other replied, "Outdated is forgivable. Inflexible is not."

"Is that what we were?"

He paused. "No. We were cautious. But caution ages faster than truth."

He moved past them slowly, struck by how gently the old guard was beginning to speak of itself.

Farther up the walkway, near the old stone terrace warmed by the day's sun, he found a pair of mid-career scholars leaning against the railing, watching a few remaining patches of frost glisten in the lamplight.

"We treated the warning as a destination instead of a waypoint," one said.

Her colleague nodded. "We froze the guidance when we should have allowed it to evolve."

"And what unfreezes a field?"

She smiled faintly. "The same thing that unfreezes a river: time and pressure."

He admired the clarity of that line — perfectly measured, perfectly true.

Outside the global exchange atrium, a wide semicircle of international researchers lingered beneath the tall lamps, their postures relaxed in ways earlier movements had not yet permitted.

A scientist from Colombia said, "Our agencies hesitated because fear was familiar."

A colleague from Finland replied, "And because familiarity felt safer than correction."

A researcher from India added, "But we've crossed the threshold now. No one wants to return to the old vocabulary."

"What replaces it?"

"Precision," she said. "Without alarm."

He walked past, recognizing that this was perhaps the most significant shift of all:

the world was not abandoning caution; it was abandoning dramatization.

Near the humanities center, a group of doctoral candidates gathered on the steps, their books stacked beside them, their conversation unfolding with the intellectual ease of people newly freed from inherited assumptions.

One said, "It's strange to think the world is correcting itself in our lifetime."

Another replied, "It's stranger to think it resisted the correction for so long."

A third added, "Fear has a long half-life."

"And truth?"

"Truth is stable," she said. "But uptake is slow."

He continued on, sensing the ground beneath him growing firmer with each passing night, each passing movement.

And then he reached the river.

Tonight, the river no longer resembled a process.

It resembled a condition.

The ice had softened into broad, translucent planes — elegant, drifting pieces that carried memory but not dominance. The water between them shimmered in wide, fluid pathways that reflected the lamps in strokes of trembling gold. The central current had widened into something unmistakable — a broad, coherent spine carrying everything forward with the authority of inevitability.

He approached the railing, and what he saw was no longer a metaphor for generations or guidance or correction.

It was a metaphor for continuity itself.

The older season — the ice — drifted with softened dignity, participating rather than resisting.

The younger season — the current — flowed with a coherence that needed no justification.

And the threshold between them — the fractures — had matured into a network of connection, not separation.

He watched as one large, softened sheet of ice tilted gently, rotated, and aligned itself with the flow, moving forward with the confidence of something that had finally stopped trying to maintain its old architecture.

The sound — that faint, crystalline brushing of ice surrendering to water — carried the unmistakable tone of release.

And standing there, he recognized something beyond the metaphor, beyond the season, beyond the narrative:

We are now fully inside the continuation.

Not approaching it.

Not preparing for it.

Not hinting at it.

Inside it.

The river is no longer changing — it is teaching.

The world is no longer resisting — it is remembering.

The research is no longer misunderstood — it is resituating itself.

The narrative is no longer building toward an ending — it is widening toward a horizon.

Nick's work extends far beyond this movement.

So does the field.

So does the global correction.

So does the intersection with Smart Gasification and environmental precision.

So does the corridor we are writing.

This is the part of the long essay where the structure becomes a landscape, and the landscape becomes a future.

He remained by the railing until the river's movement felt like part of his own breathing. Then he turned back toward the campus lights — slow, steady, assured — carrying the unmistakable knowledge that the next movement would deepen the continuity that now defined the entire work.

There were nights when the world felt both lighter and larger, as if the atmosphere itself had been rinsed clear of its earlier weight. The thaw had reached a point where even the shadows felt articulate. The lamps along the path cast long, lucid reflections across the damp pavement, and the softened earth released a faint scent—soil, bark, river moisture—reminding anyone attentive enough that the season had crossed a threshold it would not recross.

He stepped into that widened stillness.

Tonight, the campus did not resemble a place transitioning between states; it resembled a place that had accepted its new coherence. The hush in the air was not silence but agreement. Hallways glowed with softened light. Windows, once harsh with fluorescent blue, now projected a warmer tone—as if the buildings themselves understood the world had stopped arguing with itself.

Near the analytical sciences wing, he passed two senior researchers in quiet conversation.

One said, "We feared revising the guidance would undermine trust."

The other replied, "The refusal to revise is what undermines it."

"And now?"

"Now we earn trust by updating it."

He continued, feeling the relief embedded in that admission.

Farther along, near the crest of the small hill overlooking the quad, a pair of policy architects leaned against the railing, watching steam rise from the ground where the last pocket of frost had finally surrendered.

“We treated the old guidelines like a monument,” one said.

Her colleague nodded. “When they were meant to be scaffolding.”

“Doesn’t scaffolding need to come down?”

“Only after it’s been replaced.”

He admired the precision of that metaphor—gentle, truthful, necessary.

Outside the global collaboration building, a constellation of visiting scholars lingered in the lamplight, their voices carrying that calm vibration found only in people who have released a long-held tension.

A scientist from Argentina said, “For years, we mistook unanimity for accuracy.”

A colleague from Switzerland replied, “Unanimity is comfort. Accuracy is responsibility.”

A researcher from South Africa added, “Fear was the lens. Selenium changes the lens.”

Someone in the group asked, “And what does the world want now?”

“Balance,” she said. “Quiet, but firm.”

He walked past, knowing instinctively that this was where global policy would eventually land—not in drama, but in proportion.

Near the humanities concourse, a group of graduate students sat in loose circles on the steps, their discussions blending theory, ethics, and quietly radical clarity.

One said, "It feels strange to watch an entire field remake itself."

Another replied, "It feels necessary."

A third added, "It feels overdue."

"And our role?"

"To respect the correction," she said. "And to carry it forward without resentment."

He continued toward the river.

Tonight, the river no longer resembled a site of transition.

It resembled a site of memory—alive, fluid, fully engaged in its own restoration.

The ice had thinned into broad, luminous sheets that drifted with a serene confidence. The channels between them glowed with continuous movement, reflecting the lamps in wide strokes that seemed almost calligraphic. And the central current—broad, deep, authoritative—flowed with a resonance that suggested the river had finally recovered its identity.

He approached the railing.

What he saw was not a metaphor shifting.

It was a metaphor completing its purpose.

The older season — the ice — drifted with softened edges, contributing memory without obstruction.

The younger season — the current — carried everything forward with a coherence so natural it didn't need to insist upon itself.

And the place where they met — the fractures — had become the architecture of continuity.

He watched as a particularly elegant sheet of ice caught the current, rotated gently, and aligned itself with the flow—its movement so coordinated, so unforced, that it felt like witnessing a quiet intelligence at work.

The sound—a faint crystalline brushing—seemed to signal not release but resonance.

And standing there, he understood with perfect clarity:

This narrative is no longer building toward a conclusion.

It is building toward a condition.

The work has entered the phase where the pages do not close the corridor—they extend it.

Nick's research continues.

The global understanding continues.

The recalibration continues.

The integration with environmental systems continues.

Smart Gasification and biochemical clarity continue converging in quiet, elegant ways the world is only beginning to articulate.

Continuation is now the grammar of the essay.

He remained at the railing until the river's movement synced with the rhythm of the night, then turned toward the campus—the lights steady, the pathways assured—ready to guide the reader deeper into the widening continuity.

There were nights when the world felt almost over-attentive, as though the air itself had leaned in to listen. The temperature had settled into that rare equilibrium where nothing pleaded for change — not the soil beneath the walkway, not the half-thawed grass, not the river's slow articulation of its widening channels. Even the lamps seemed to cast their light less urgently, as if illumination had become a natural byproduct rather than an effort.

He stepped into that attentive calm.

Tonight, the campus carried the unmistakable sensation of a place that had begun to grasp its own trajectory. Not in a declarative sense — there were no announcements, no banners, no visible shifts — but in the quiet, instinctive way a landscape knows when winter has truly lost its claim.

Near the policy coordination building, he passed two senior advisors standing under a vaulted awning, their breath faint in the cooling air.

One said, "For years we mistook rigidity for responsibility."

The other replied, "Responsibility is flexible. Rigidity is fear."

"And the public?"

"They're ahead of us. They've been ahead for a while."

He continued, noting how their tone had abandoned defensiveness. This was no longer a conversation about justification. It was a conversation about maturation.

Farther along the walkway, near a cluster of still-damp stone benches, a pair of researchers stood watching the gentle dissolution of a remaining frost patch.

"We believed we were shielding pregnant women from risk," one said.

Her colleague answered softly, "And we were shielding ourselves from revision."

"We thought the narrative was settled."

"The narrative was comfortable," he said. "And comfort is a powerful blindfold."

He recognized the importance in the softness of their voices — not regret, but dawning clarity.

Outside the international symposium hall, a broad group of delegates remained in a loosely formed circle, each speaking with the measured cadence of someone who had thought deeply before offering an opinion.

A scholar from Peru said, "Our communities embraced the science long before our agencies did."

A researcher from Norway replied, "Our agencies clung to caution because caution was predictable."

A fellow from Japan added, "Predictability became habit. And habit became doctrine."

A voice from Kenya asked, "And what replaces doctrine when its time ends?"

The Peruvian scholar considered this. “Practice,” she said. “Simply... better practice.”

He passed them quietly, struck by how rarely global agreement arrived through force — and how often through exhaustion of the old.

Near the humanities steps, groups of graduate students gathered in quiet clusters, not frantic or burdened, but reflective, as though they understood the significance of living through a period that was already becoming historical.

One said, “We’re the first generation who won’t inherit the old warning unaltered.”

Another replied, “We’ll inherit the correction instead.”

A third added, “Our job is to keep the correction alive long enough to become culture.”

“And culture?”

“Culture is simply clarity that has survived repetition.”

He continued toward the river, sensing the landscape anticipates him now — not because he is different, but because the world around him is beginning to speak more softly, more precisely.

The river waited.

Tonight, the river displayed not transition, not thaw, not even arrival — but integration.

A stage past metaphor, past symbol, past instructional clarity.

This was the river in the full expression of its new season.

The ice had softened into broad, luminous islands that drifted with the fragile confidence of something learning to trust the current that carries it. The pathways between these islands had widened into elegant, uninterrupted corridors of water, shimmering beneath lamp reflections in long, patient ribbons. And the central current — wide, resonant, assured — moved with the quiet authority of something that had been waiting for this moment all winter.

He approached the railing.

What he saw now was not the relationship between generations, nor between science and fear, nor between institutions and their corrections.

What he saw was the truth of long work.

The older season — the ice — no longer resisted, no longer hesitated, no longer clung to its old geometry. It drifted with dignity, memory intact, authority surrendered.

The younger season — the current — did not gloat, did not hurry, did not overwhelm. It flowed with a natural coherence that needed nothing affirmed.

And the threshold — the fractures — had refined themselves into connective tissue, elegant transitions, the architecture through which continuity expressed itself.

He watched as a broad sheet of ice slid into the main channel, rotated slowly, and merged fully with the river's forward movement. The sound of softened ice brushing against water felt less like release now and more like recognition.

And standing there, he understood:

We are no longer approaching the continuation.

We are inhabiting it.

The field continues.

Nick's work continues.

Public understanding continues.

Institutional recalibration continues.

Environmental clarity — from fisheries to Smart Gasification — continues.

The narrative continues.

The river teaches by flowing, not by concluding.

He stood there until the night softened into its own kind of coherence, then turned from the railing and began walking back toward the campus lights — the corridor widening behind him, around him, within him — ready to receive the next movement, not as extension, but as belonging.

There were nights when the air carried a different sort of intelligence — not the sharp, bracing intellect of winter, and not the eager, restless intellect of spring, but something slower, older, more contemplative. The kind of intelligence that comes from systems learning how to breathe together after a long season of discord. The lamps glowed with a steadiness that felt earned, not assumed. Their light stretched farther across the softened earth, as though illumination itself had gained confidence.

He stepped into that contemplative intelligence.

Tonight, the campus had the atmosphere of a place practicing its future.

Not deciding it.

Not defending it.

Practicing it.

Near the environmental sciences annex, two senior faculty members stood in conversation under a modest overhang, their voices hushed but free of tension.

One said, “We thought rigidity kept us safe.”

The other replied, “It only kept us static.”

“And static systems?”

“Collapse,” she said. “They always collapse under their own memory.”

He walked past them, recognizing that this was not bitterness speaking — it was wisdom finally freed from its own hesitation.

A little farther on, near a shallow pool where meltwater had gathered, he saw two research fellows studying the reflection of the lamps.

“We underestimated the public’s capacity for proportion,” one said.

Her colleague nodded. “And overestimated their appetite for fear.”

“What replaces fear when its season ends?”

“Interpretation,” he answered. “And interpretation is quieter.”

He carried that thought with him like a narrowed beam of light.

Outside the global public health center, a cluster of international researchers lingered in the broad circle of lamplight, speaking in measured voices that suggested not debate, but alignment.

A physician from Malaysia said, “Our guidance clung to an era that didn’t survive its own evidence.”

A colleague from Denmark replied, “Our ministries feared the optics of admitting that.”

A researcher from Uruguay added, “But the optics of delay are worse.”

A scientist from Morocco tilted her head. “What finally overcame the resistance?”

“Time,” she said softly. “And the quiet insistence of data.”

He understood immediately: truth rarely arrives loudly, but it persists.

Near the humanities steps, a cluster of graduate students leaned against the stone columns, their expressions lit by a confidence unburdened by the anxieties of the previous generation.

One said, “We don’t see the correction as controversial.”

Another replied, “We see it as overdue.”

A third added, “We were taught to trust proportion, not panic.”

“And to question inherited frameworks,” someone said.

“That’s what makes us different,” she answered. “We weren’t raised in fear.”

He passed them, sensing that this — this generational ease — was the true signal of a shift becoming permanent.

The night deepened as he approached the river.

Tonight, the river looked less like a place and more like a verdict — not a harsh one, not punitive, but an evolutionary verdict, the kind water reaches when it has outlasted every resistance placed in its path.

The ice had thinned into broad, translucent sheets that floated with the composure of things no longer pretending to control their fate. The channels between them glimmered like open corridors — wide, patient, precise. And the central current flowed with an authority that no longer needed to assert itself. It simply carried the world forward.

He reached the railing.

What the river showed him tonight was not thaw.

Not transition.

Not even integration.

It showed him inheritance.

The older season — the ice — continued to drift, softened, humbled, not erased, remembered.

The younger season — the current — continued to widen its path, not aggressively, not triumphantly, but steadily, like truth taking its rightful place.

And the fractures — once symbols of rupture — now resembled tributaries of knowledge, guiding the last remnants of winter into the logic of the new season.

He watched a particularly large sheet of ice turn gently, then glide into the main channel, moving with a dignity that felt almost ceremonial. The sound — that familiar crystalline whisper — carried the tone of a world adjusting to the knowledge it could no longer defer.

And he understood something deeper now, something the river had been preparing him to recognize:

We have crossed the threshold where the continuation is not a future chapter —

it is the present condition.

Nick's work continues beyond the page.

Institutional recalibration continues beyond the page.

Public reorientation continues beyond the page.

The intersection with Smart Gasification continues beyond the page.

Environmental sovereignty continues beyond the page.

Clarity continues beyond the page.

The page is no longer the boundary.

It is the witness.

He remained by the railing until the river's cadence aligned with the cadence of the night, then turned back toward the campus — walking with the quiet authority of someone who knows that the next movement will deepen the continuity that now defines everything.

There were nights when the world seemed to expand without moving — when the atmosphere took on a depth that felt almost architectural, as though the air itself had stepped forward to reveal a structure it had been holding in reserve. The temperature hovered at a perfect equilibrium: cool enough to quiet the mind, warm enough to loosen the breath. The lamps along the walkways cast smooth, unwavering ellipses of gold across the damp ground, and the softened earth carried the scent of renewal rising from below the surface.

He stepped into that spacious equilibrium.

Tonight, the campus had the composure of a place no longer discussing transformation, but inhabiting it. The rhythm of footsteps was slower, more deliberate. Conversations drifted with the calm cadence of people who had finally stopped bracing for contradiction. Even the buildings seemed lighter — less burdened by the centuries of institutional caution they had inherited.

Near the faculty governance wing, he passed two seasoned administrators speaking beneath a modest canopy.

One said, “We clung to the old paradigm because it felt reliable.”

The other replied, “Reliability is an illusion when the premise is outdated.”

“And reliability gave us cover.”

She shook her head. “Cover is not the same as clarity.”

He continued, sensing that this was the precise moment when institutions begin to tell the truth to themselves.

Further up the path, near a cluster of benches made slick by melting frost, two mid-grade researchers paused to observe the sheen of water forming along the walkway.

“We called it uncertainty,” one said.

Her colleague exhaled softly. “It was fear disguised as uncertainty.”

“Fear of being wrong?”

“Fear of revising ourselves.”

He carried that with him — the recognition that revision is not a threat, but a task.

Outside the global health pavilion, a constellation of scholars spoke in low voices, their shoulders relaxed in the lamplit quiet.

A fellow from Spain said, “Our doctors resisted because the narrative was easier to maintain than to correct.”

A scientist from Vietnam replied, “Narratives are comfortable. Corrections are lonely.”

A colleague from Canada added, “But loneliness is a temporary cost.”

A researcher from Senegal nodded. “Truth has no cost once the world accepts it.”

He walked past, hearing in their voices the slow dissolution of the old orthodoxy.

Near the arts and humanities building, a group of graduate students leaned against the stone columns, speaking with the effortless confidence of those who have grown up without the burden of inherited fear.

One said, “It’s strange: our entire generation defaults to the newer framework.”

Another replied, “Because proportion feels familiar to us.”

A third added, “Fear feels foreign.”

“And foreignness fades when truth becomes habitual.”

He continued, aware of how seamlessly the younger generation had stepped into alignment with clarity.

And then he approached the river.

Tonight, the river had settled into its fullest expression — the stage of the season where transition becomes identity.

The ice had softened into broad, translucent masses that drifted with the quiet self-awareness of things no longer pretending to resist. The pathways of water between them had widened into stately corridors—fluid, shimmering, almost ceremonial. And the central current flowed with a coherence that felt less like motion and more like inheritance.

He stepped to the railing.

Tonight, the river revealed the architecture of long work:

The older season — ice — no longer defined the structure; it contributed to it.

The younger season — water — no longer argued with the remnants of winter; it absorbed them.

And the fractures — once the language of conflict — had become the grammar of integration.

He watched as a wide sheet of softened ice slid into the main channel, its edges catching the lamplight, turning gently before merging into the inevitable movement of the river. The soft brushing sound that followed carried a new resonance — not release, not surrender, but recognition.

And he understood:

We are fully within the widening now.

The essay is no longer reaching for continuation.

It is continuation.

Nick's work extends through this moment.

His research advances in ways neither the old narrative nor the earlier science could contain.

The global correction continues its slow, steady recalibration.

Environmental clarity — from fish physiology to atmospheric chemistry to Smart Gasification — continues to converge in a single, widening frame.

The reader has crossed into a world where the pages are not boundaries but thresholds.

He remained at the railing until the river's rhythm synchronized with the night, then turned back toward the campus lights — walking not toward a conclusion, but toward the next widening, the next deepening, the next articulation of a world that has learned to move without fear.

There were mornings — and they were always mornings, never afternoons — when Nick arrived at the podium carrying the same quiet certainty he carried into the lab. A certainty not of triumph or persuasion, but of continuity. The kind of certainty that comes from doing the same work for so long that the world's resistance no longer feels like opposition, but like climate.

The auditorium always smelled faintly of old carpet and new technology. There were placards neatly arranged on each chair, the logo of whatever conference was hosting him printed in crisp colors that did nothing to disguise the fact that half the audience still believed mercury was the villain of the story.

He stepped to the podium.

He didn't rush.

He never rushed.

Rushing belonged to the people who were afraid of being questioned.

Nick had long since outgrown that fear.

He clicked the first slide.

A biochemical pathway illuminated the screen — selenium metabolism at its most elegant, the cascade of enzymes, the interplay of oxidative pressure, the delicate choreography of binding sites and protective ratios. The diagram glowed softly, as though the molecular world were offering its own quiet testimony.

He began.

Not with urgency.

Not with persuasion.

But with clarity that had been honed by thousands of repetitions across two decades.

“Selenium,” he said in that gentle, measured voice, “is not optional. It is essential.”

A few heads nodded.

A few remained still.

Several young researchers scribbled notes, though they didn’t need to — they already knew the framework.

He advanced the slide.

The next diagram showed the deactivation pathways — how mercury, unbound, can interfere with selenium-dependent enzymes, and how selenium, in sufficient presence, protects the developing brain from precisely that interruption.

It was the slide that always divided a room.

He could feel it happen again:

A quarter of the audience leaned forward — curious, open, ready.

Another half remained neutral — processing, recalibrating, cautious but not dismissive.

And the final quarter stiffened imperceptibly — the long shadow of the old warning tightening its grip.

He had seen that posture in every country, every language, every funding cycle.

It never rattled him.

It merely told him where he needed to begin.

He continued.

His cadence shifted slightly when he spoke of the fetus — not softer, not louder, just more deliberate. The brain's development, the dependence on omega-3s, the reliance on selenoenzymes, the protective ratios that had been misunderstood for decades. The entire sequence felt like watching a craftsman reveal the grain of a material others had mistaken for something else.

Then came the objections.

They always came.

Sometimes whispered.

Sometimes spoken aloud.

Sometimes disguised as questions.

Occasionally disguised as compliments.

This time it was a woman in the third row — a mid-career nutritionist who had lived under the old paradigm long enough to feel its removal as a kind of betrayal.

"But how can we tell the public they were mistaken?" she asked.

Nick paused.

Not out of hesitation.

Out of respect — not for the question, but for the fear behind it.

"We're not telling them they were mistaken," he said. "We're telling them the science has matured."

A subtle distinction.

But a necessary one.

He clicked to the next slide — the long dataset, the international comparison, the deep ocean species lined up against their selenium-to-mercury profiles. The truth was right there — crystalline, measurable, reproducible — yet the room was still warming to it by degrees.

That had always been the challenge:

fear introduced the story,

so fear felt entitled to conclude it.

But Nick did not conclude stories.

He corrected them.

The questions continued.

"What about high-mercury fish?"

"What about public perception?"

"What about liability?"

"What about the old advisories?"

"What about the agencies that endorsed them?"

"What about countries that still teach the outdated model?"

"What about pediatricians?"

"What about the media?"

Nick answered each with patience, not persuasion:

"Look at the ratios."

"Look at the protective thresholds."

"Look at the enzymatic functions."

"Look at the population outcomes."

"Look at the consistency across species."

"Look at the cost of perpetuating fear."

"Look at the biochemical truth."

Truth, in his hands, was never adversarial.

It was simply inevitable.

He watched the room soften — not agree, not convert, not capitulate — but soften. The first step in any correction is not acceptance; it is softening. The unfreezing of intellectual posture.

When his presentation ended, the applause was polite, restrained, thoughtful. Not triumphant. Not dismissive.

He didn't need triumph.

He needed continuity.

As people filtered out of the auditorium, a few approached him — younger researchers, early-career physicians, graduate students. Their questions were precise, curious, unburdened by the old fear. They weren't fighting a paradigm; they were inheriting a correction.

Nick smiled the small, quiet smile of a man who has been doing this so long that progress feels like weather — unpredictable in any moment, but inevitable across seasons.

He gathered his materials, closed his laptop, and walked toward the exit.

Outside, the campus air was still cool, but no longer cold.

The thaw was no longer metaphor.

It was context.

And his work — the long, slow, elegant correction — moved with him into the night.

There were afternoons when the real work didn't happen in auditoriums or advisory board rooms at all, but in the places no one ever photographs: the narrow labs where the hum of equipment becomes a kind of second heartbeat, or the quiet wings of the university where fluorescence pools against tile floors and the hours pass unnoticed.

These were the places where his persistence took shape.

Today it happened in the lab.

Not the main lab — that one hosted tours, visiting dignitaries, grant reviewers.

This was the side lab, the one tucked behind the larger research suite, where instruments had been calibrated so many times they carried the faint scent of ethanol and memory.

He stood over the workstation, reviewing a set of bioassay results with one of the postdocs — a sharp, steady researcher who had joined the team precisely because she sensed the work was larger than its reception.

“Here,” she said, tapping the screen with a gloved finger. “The selenium-binding curve is exactly where we expected.”

“And the mercury inhibition?” he asked.

She zoomed in on the graph, her expression tightening, then relaxing.

“Lower,” she said. “Meaning the protective enzymes aren’t being disrupted at this concentration.”

He nodded.

This was the kind of evidence he had built his career upon:

not dramatic findings, not spectacular revelations, but the cumulative refinement of the truth — measured, reproducible, consistent.

Yet even here, in the place where science should have been immune to narrative, the questions found him.

Another researcher leaned into the doorway.

“Can I ask something?” she said. “Why does the messaging lag so far behind the data?”

He didn’t answer immediately.

He never rushed these questions.

They were honest questions, not challenges.

Finally he said, "Because the original warning was moralized. And moral narratives are hard to replace with biochemical ones."

She folded her arms. "But the evidence is clear."

"Yes," he said softly. "But clarity is slow when fear arrives first."

The postdoc looked up from the screen.

"Do you ever wonder what would've happened if you hadn't pushed this for twenty years?"

He smiled — that small, understated smile that appeared only when questions touched the deeper layers of his work.

"I didn't push it," he said. "The data did."

The postdoc laughed under her breath. "You carried it."

He shook his head gently.

"I clarified it."

But the truth — unspoken, understood — was this:

He carried the burden of correction long before anyone else wanted to.

Later that day, he sat in his office, surrounded by half-processed manuscripts, printed datasets, and three versions of a policy brief marked with quiet editorial scars:

language softened,

terms adjusted,

phrasing reshaped for palatability.

He leaned back in his chair, studying one particular sentence:

"Selenium may mitigate the neurodevelopmental risk previously attributed solely to mercury."

The sentence was cautious.

Careful.

Gentle.

It was the kind of sentence a reviewer would accept.

It was also the kind of sentence that underrepresented the truth.

He picked up a pen and — without irritation, without theatrics — crossed out the word may.

Clarity, even at its quietest, demanded accuracy.

He replaced it with:

"Selenium protects the developing brain from mercury-induced enzyme disruption."

Direct.

Precise.

Scientifically uncontroversial.

Politically inconvenient.

He set the draft aside, knowing it would raise eyebrows among reviewers who preferred softer language — not because the science was uncertain, but because certainty made people uncomfortable when it threatened old frameworks.

He didn't resent the discomfort.

He simply refused to center it.

That evening, as the last of the faculty filtered out and the hallways fell quiet, he walked toward the river — not for symbolism but for habit. The walk helped him think. The landscape offered rhythm. The water offered proportion.

The river had reached its newest stage:

the softened ice drifting in slow procession, the channels widening, the current carrying the season forward without hesitation.

He leaned on the railing, the cold metal steady under his hands.

This was the part no one saw:

not the conferences,

not the advisory rooms,

not the global forums.

This — the clarity settling in the mind after a full day of work — was the true cost of scientific persistence.

The river didn't reassure him.

It aligned with him.

The season didn't congratulate him.

It contextualized him.

His work didn't resolve anything.

It continued.

He closed his eyes briefly, listening to the soft, crystalline brushing of ice drifting along the surface.

It sounded almost like the world learning.

There were mornings when the objections arrived before the coffee had finished brewing.

Not hostile objections — those were mostly gone now.

Not ideological objections — those had faded with the old guard.

These were the residual objections, the ones shaped by habit, by muscle memory, by the echo of a warning repeated long enough to become cultural.

He had come to expect them.

He had even come to understand them.

Today's came in the form of an email sent at 6:47 a.m. from a regional clinical director — a well-meaning professional who had built an entire career around advising pregnant mothers to avoid fish.

The subject line read:

"A question about risk communication."

Nick opened it.

The message was polite, thoughtful, concerned.

If we tell women now that fish is beneficial,

won't they accuse us of misleading them before?

What happens when public trust is shaken?

How do we revise a guideline that became identity for so many clinicians?

He read it twice.

Not because he doubted the answer —

but because he respected the fear in the question.

Fear always reveals itself when the truth begins to move.

He typed a response slowly, deliberately:

"We are not reversing course.

We are correcting course.

Correction is not contradiction — it is maturation."

He added nothing more.

Nothing less was needed.

Later that day, he attended a virtual panel hosted by a national health coalition.

The faces arranged themselves into neat rectangles across the screen:

pediatricians, nutritionists, epidemiologists, policy advisors, environmental scientists.

These were good people —

smart, earnest, well-intentioned —

but many of them still lived inside the vocabulary of the old paradigm.

A pediatrician unmuted herself.

“I understand the biochemical model,” she said carefully, “but I’m afraid the public won’t.”

Nick nodded gently.

“Then we simplify,” he said. “Without distorting.”

“But how do we simplify without downplaying risk?” she asked.

“We don’t downplay risk,” he replied. “We contextualize it.”

A fisheries biologist added, “Context is harder to communicate than fear.”

Nick’s expression softened.

“Fear is simple because it’s incomplete,” he said.

“Context is harder because it’s accurate.”

A policy strategist leaned forward toward the camera.

“Do you really believe the field is ready to shift?” he asked.

Nick didn’t rush.

He never rushed these moments.

“The field is already shifting,” he said. “The question is whether the guidance wants to follow.”

There was a long silence —

not discomfort, but recognition.

These were the moments where clarity landed.

Not with applause or argument,

but with the soft weight of inevitability.

When the meeting ended, he walked down the hallway toward his office, but was stopped by a young researcher leaning against the wall — a graduate student he remembered from a symposium last spring.

She held a notebook close to her chest.

"Can I ask a naïve question?" she said.

"There are no naïve questions," he replied.

"Then... why did the warning last so long?" she asked.

"We've had the data for years."

He smiled faintly.

"Because the first story people hear is the hardest one to unlearn."

She nodded, absorbing that.

"But you kept correcting it," she said.

"Because the second story," he replied, "is the one that lasts."

She looked down at her notebook, as though trying to capture the sentence before it slipped away.

He walked on.

Later, in the lab, he reviewed a new dataset — fresh results from a coastal study. The selenium levels in the sampled populations were robust. Mercury levels were low. The protective ratios held across age groups.

He felt no triumph.

Only confirmation.

The kind of confirmation that arrives like steady rain —

quiet, continuous, undeniable.

A colleague stepped into the room.

"Did you see the new analysis?" she asked.

"It matches the model almost perfectly."

He nodded.

"The models have been right for a long time," he said.

"We're just catching up."

She hesitated.

"Do you ever get tired?"

He smiled — not broadly, just enough for the truth to show.

"I get tired," he said. "But the work doesn't."

And the room fell into a silence shaped not by fatigue, but by continuity — the kind of silence that carries the weight of decades, softened by the knowledge that the correction is finally gathering momentum.

That evening, he walked once more toward the river.

Tonight, the river did not resemble thaw or transition or even arrival.

It resembled persistence — the quiet, unbroken movement of a system that understands its direction and does not need to accelerate.

The softened ice drifted in broad, luminous sheets.

The channels shimmered in slow, articulate motion.

The current carried everything with a calm authority that did not need to prove anything to anyone.

He stood at the railing, listening to the familiar crystalline brushing of ice against water.

It sounded like repetition.

It sounded like correction.

It sounded like a story finally learning to rewrite itself.

There were conferences that felt more like crossroads than events — not because of the agenda, not because of the venue, but because of the kinds of questions that surfaced when people realized the old paradigm was no longer enough to carry them.

This one took place in a coastal city, in a conference center built almost entirely of glass. The ocean glimmered behind the speakers' silhouettes, as though the water itself were listening.

Nick stood at the edge of the room, not hiding, not performing — simply observing. He always observed before he spoke. It was part of his method: let the temperature of the room reveal itself before attempting to correct its climate.

Today, the temperature was conflicted.

On one side:

younger researchers, eager, unburdened by decades of inherited fear.

On the other:

seasoned clinicians whose reputations had been built on warnings now eroding under the pressure of biochemical truth.

Between them:

a wide middle, unsure which story would define the next decade.

The panel moderator introduced him, and he walked to the stage without hurry.

He didn't project authority.

Authority projected him.

The first question came almost immediately, from a senior clinician whose voice carried the firmness of someone accustomed to being right.

"Dr. Ralston, with respect—how do you reconcile your findings with decades of public health advisories? Those advisories shaped whole generations of maternal guidelines. Are you saying they were wrong?"

He didn't flinch.

"I'm saying they were based on the best model we had at the time."

A murmur passed through the room — relief for some, discomfort for others.

He continued:

"But models evolve.

Data accumulates.

Truth refines.

Science matures."

The clinician leaned forward.

"That sounds like revision."

Nick shook his head gently.

"It's not revision," he said.

"It's completion."

The room stilled.

Completion —

a word that honored the past without awarding it the final chapter.

The next question came from a public health advisor who looked young enough to still believe the world could be corrected without resistance.

"Why didn't the agencies update their guidance sooner?" she asked.

Nick held her gaze with the soft steadiness that had become his signature.

"Because guidance moves at the speed of consensus," he said. "Not at the speed of truth."

A quiet ripple of recognition spread through the room.

Someone in the back whispered, "He's right," and didn't bother to hide it.

Then came the question he always expected — the one that revealed the real obstacle.

A nutrition organization representative raised her hand.

"If we adopt your framework now," she said carefully, "how do we communicate it without undermining public trust? It feels risky to say we've changed our position."

He nodded slowly.

"It's not risky," he said.

"It's honest."

"But the public may think we misled them," she insisted.

He paused.

When he answered, the entire room leaned in slightly, as if the air itself had asked for the clarification.

"We didn't mislead them," he said.

"We protected them with the information we had."

"And now?" she asked.

"Now," he said, "we protect them with better information."

A few heads bowed in quiet agreement — not conversion, not capitulation, but acceptance of a season that had already changed.

During the break, a group of young researchers gathered around him.

One asked, "Do you think the old paradigm will disappear completely?"

He smiled — a patient, knowing smile, the kind shaped by twenty-five years of explaining the same molecular truth to rooms that shifted only by inches at a time.

"No paradigm disappears," he said. "It simply becomes unnecessary."

"And then?" someone asked.

"Then the new one becomes obvious."

They scribbled that down, though it didn't need to be written.

It would echo in them for years.

Later, as the day's sessions wound down and the coastal fog drifted across the glass facade, he walked outside toward the water.

The ocean looked almost metallic in the diffuse light — a vast, quiet ledger holding the biochemical truth of the world's fish populations, indifferent to politics, immune to bureaucracy, endlessly patient with human misunderstanding.

He watched a wave break gently along the shoreline.

The ocean had always known the correction.

It had always held the truth.

It had never once changed the way it behaved.

He stood there, listening to the tide as though it were a familiar colleague.

And in that moment, he felt it again — not triumph, not fatigue, but the quiet certainty of a man whose work continued without permission, without resistance, without hurry.

The world would shift.

Slowly.

Incompletely.

Inevitably.

And when it did, it would do so not because of persuasion, but because the biochemical truth had outlived the fear.

There were symposiums where the science felt secondary to the psychology — where the real work wasn't conducted in the data sessions or the poster halls, but in the subtle way a room of experts negotiated its own discomfort.

This one was held inland, far from any coastline, in a city whose relationship to seafood was almost entirely academic. It made the conversations both clearer and stranger: clearer because no one had direct economic interest; stranger because everyone carried inherited assumptions about fish despite living a thousand miles from saltwater.

Nick sat in the second row during the keynote. The speaker — a respected environmental toxicologist —

was presenting a cautious, familiar narrative. Mercury. Exposure. Vulnerability. Warnings.

Nothing inaccurate.

Just incomplete.

Nick listened without correction, without interruption. He had learned long ago that interruption hardens positions. Correction requires timing, not volume.

When the keynote ended, the panel convened. Questions flowed predictably: exposure pathways, trophic levels, bioaccumulation patterns. Then the moderator turned to him.

"Dr. Ralston, would you like to comment on the interaction between mercury toxicity and dietary variables?"

A polite invitation.

A careful phrasing.

A subtle handoff.

He rose.

A quiet ripple moved through the room — not anticipation, not tension, something more like the soundless shift of people bracing for a reframing they weren't sure they were ready for.

He began not with data, but with proportion.

"In most of our discussions," he said, "we treat mercury as an isolated threat. We very rarely ask what it displaces in the biochemical system."

The moderator leaned forward.

A few pens stopped mid-note.

He continued:

“Toxicity isn’t just about presence. It’s about interruption.”

He clicked to his slide — a simple graphic, no color, no theatrics — illustrating the selenium-dependent enzymes in neurodevelopment.

“Selenium,” he said, “is not a nutrient in this context. It is infrastructure.”

A few eyebrows lifted.

Someone whispered, “Interesting...”

Someone else whispered, “Wait—what does he mean by infrastructure?”

He advanced the model slowly, as though unspooling a thread they had assumed was rope.

“This framework doesn’t deny mercury’s potential harm,” he said. “It contextualizes it. Mercury disrupts selenoenzymes. Selenium prevents that disruption. So the question is no longer: ‘How much mercury is present?’ The question is: ‘Is there enough selenium available to maintain neuroprotection?’”

A senior toxicologist raised his hand.

“But mercury exposure is still dangerous.”

Nick nodded.

“Yes,” he said. “When selenium is insufficient.”

The room shifted again — another subtle redistribution of understanding.

“And seafood?” another attendee asked.

“Selenium-rich,” he said. “And consistently so across species.”

A long silence followed — the kind that appears only when people realize they have been analyzing the wrong axis.

The moderator finally spoke.

“This reframes our entire risk model.”

Nick offered a small, almost apologetic smile.

“It completes it,” he said.

During the lunch break, the room reorganized itself into clusters of conversation. Some approached him directly — eager, open, energized by clarity. Others kept their distance — processing, recalibrating.

One researcher approached with a tray she’d barely touched.

“Can I ask you something?” she said. “Why didn’t I hear this earlier in my career?”

He met her gaze kindly.

“You did,” he said. “You just didn’t hear it yet.”

She stood there, absorbing that — the difference between information delivered and information received.

Later that afternoon, a breakout session focused on maternal nutrition. The panelists revisited the old warnings, the familiar guidance, the entrenched caution.

A policymaker asked him, “Do you worry about confusing the public?”

“No,” he said. “I worry about confusing the science.”

Another asked, “How long until this becomes mainstream understanding?”

He considered that for a moment.

“Scientific truth moves slowly,” he said. “But it does move.”

The moderator leaned in.

“And when it finally arrives?”

Nick gave a small shrug — not dismissive, but almost contemplative.

“By then,” he said, “it will feel obvious.”

A pause.

Not disagreement.

Recognition.

That evening, while others attended the networking reception, he slipped out the back of the conference center and walked along a quiet riverfront trail. The water here was narrower, quicker, reflecting the dusk in streaks of silver and slate.

He paused on a footbridge.

Everything in the landscape — the water, the wind, the dimming sky — felt like a continuation of the same conversation he had been having for decades.

He didn't need the river to mirror his work.

He needed it to measure it.

And it did.

Not by what had changed,

but by what had finally begun to loosen.

Above him, the first evening star emerged faintly through the thinning light.

He watched it without urgency.

Correction, he knew, was not a surge.

It was a tide.

And tides always return.

There were institutions — entire institutions — that behaved like organisms: slow to awaken, slow to pivot, slow to recognize what their own internal metabolism had already begun to accept. Nick understood this better than anyone. He knew that science progressed through individuals, but policy progressed through inertia.

Today's meeting was with one of those organisms.

A federal agency — not hostile, not obstructive, simply... anchored. Anchored to its past advisories, anchored to the narrative it had helped shape, anchored to the vocabulary it had repeated for thirty years.

They met in a conference room whose walls were lined with framed posters of past public health campaigns. Slogans that once felt protective now felt simplistic. The air had that bureaucratic stillness familiar to all government buildings — as though the room needed permission to change.

Nick sat at the long, polished table. Across from him, four senior officials reviewed a briefing packet with the cautious reverence of people handling documents that might force them to revise their own posture.

One of them — a director with decades in the field — placed her glasses on the table and exhaled slowly.

"Dr. Ralston," she said, "we understand your findings. Truly. But changing guidance requires unanimity across departments. That takes time."

He nodded.

"I understand."

"And if the new model contradicts our earlier messaging," she continued, "the public may lose trust."

He considered her carefully — her sincerity, her hesitation, her fear.

"Trust isn't lost by correction," he said. "Trust is lost by refusing to correct."

Another official leaned forward.

"But the optics—"

He stopped him gently with a raised hand.

"Optics follow truth," he said. "Not the other way around."

A long silence.

No tension.

Just the sound of an institution testing its own weight.

Finally, the youngest person in the room — a man barely in his thirties, newly promoted and still carrying the idealism of someone not yet worn down — spoke up.

“May I say something?”

The director nodded.

He turned to Nick.

“I read your research in grad school,” he said quietly. “It changed the way I think about nutrition. I’ve been waiting years for this agency to catch up.”

The older officials stiffened slightly — not offended, just surprised.

Nick gave a small nod — a gesture that acknowledged both gratitude and recognition.

“It will catch up,” he said softly. “But only if the science is allowed to lead.”

The young official inhaled, steadying himself.

“Then we should lead with clarity,” he said.

No one responded immediately.

But something subtle in the room loosened — the faintest release of institutional tension, as though a first hinge had finally shifted.

When the meeting adjourned, a deputy asked to walk with him down the hallway.

She spoke in a low voice.

“You know,” she said, “half of my colleagues worry that if we rewrite the guideline, it will imply they were negligent before. They’re afraid of owning that.”

Nick slowed his steps.

“They don’t have to own negligence,” he said. “They only have to own growth.”

She looked at him, startled by the simplicity of it.

“And the public?” she asked.

“The public,” he said, “is more forgiving than institutions expect — as long as we tell the truth plainly.”

They reached the elevator.

She hesitated before stepping inside.

“So... you believe the shift is inevitable?” she asked.

He offered the faintest smile.

“Inevitable,” he said, “is a biochemical term long before it’s a policy term.”

The elevator doors closed.

Later that afternoon, he walked back across campus as the wind carried loose snow in delicate spirals across the pavement. The buildings rose around him in shades of winter white and muted steel, the familiar geography of decades of work.

A graduate student hurried to catch up with him.

"Dr. Ralston!" she called out, her breath visible in the air. "I read your latest correspondence with the agency. Are they really considering updating the guidelines?"

He nodded gently.

"They're considering considering it," he said.

She laughed softly.

"That sounds about right."

He stopped at the corner of the building, watching the snow drift along the sidewalk.

"Change is like this," he said quietly. "Not a storm — a slow accumulation."

She followed his gaze.

"But the science is clear," she said. "Why isn't that enough?"

He answered without looking away from the drifting snow.

"Because clarity moves at one speed," he said. "And consensus moves at another."

"And which one wins?"

"Clarity," he said. "Always clarity. It just takes longer."

That evening, as he left the building for the long walk toward the river, the sky was thick with overcast light — a pale, soft gray that dissolved the horizon. Everything felt suspended: the air, the snow, the season itself.

The world around him was neither winter nor spring.

It was the in-between.

The place where change is happening even when no one sees it.

He stopped at the riverbank.

The surface was a mosaic of drifting floes — fragments of ice moving in slow, considered motion. Not breaking. Not forming. Just... changing.

He watched them drift, each one carrying the quiet message he had lived his whole career:

Correction is slow.

Correction is steady.

Correction is certain.

And when the world finally recognizes it, the recognition will feel like something that had been true all along.

There were committees whose very design made them allergic to urgency. Committees that moved like glaciers — wide, heavy, slow — not because the people lacked intelligence, but because the structure itself rewarded hesitation. Nick understood this. He had never faulted them for moving slowly; he only faulted them when they mistook slowness for prudence.

Today, he met with one of the largest of these committees.

Thirty members.

Four subcommittees.

Three layers of review.

One mission: to evaluate emerging scientific consensus in maternal nutrition.

They met in a vaulted conference auditorium that looked more like an old lecture hall retrofitted with new screens. The chairs were arranged in concentric arcs, allowing everyone to see everyone else — a design choice that unintentionally encouraged both boldness and avoidance.

Nick sat quietly at the center table.

A thick binder lay in front of each committee member — hundreds of pages of data, charts, enzymatic pathways, population studies, risk analyses, all leading toward a single conclusion that had taken twenty-five years to articulate properly:

The model was ready to change.

But readiness was never the problem.

Acceptance was.

The chair of the committee cleared her throat.

"Dr. Ralston," she said, "thank you for your patience. Our internal review team has prepared some questions."

Patience.

The word lingered in the air like a polite apology.

He nodded.

A senior member raised his hand. His hair was silver, his posture rigid, his voice shaped by decades of authority.

“Our current guidelines emphasize mercury risk in pregnancy. If we shift to emphasize selenium’s protective role, how do we prevent misinterpretation?”

Nick answered with quiet precision:

“We don’t prevent misinterpretation. We prevent distortion. Misinterpretation corrects itself when given time. Distortion survives by design.”

A few committee members exchanged glances — the kind that indicate they had not expected the argument to be so clean.

Another member leaned forward.

“But the public trusts the warnings we’ve given for thirty years. They might feel betrayed if we change course.”

Nick folded his hands.

“The public,” he said softly, “trusts clarity more than consistency.”

A murmur rippled across the rows.

Not disagreement — recognition.

The kind of recognition that occurs when someone articulates something everyone knows privately but fears saying aloud.

A younger member — mid-thirties, energetic, earnest — asked:

"What does the data actually show about neurodevelopment outcomes when fish is avoided entirely during pregnancy?"

Nick's expression softened.

"Developmental deficits," he said.

"Consistently."

She nodded, scribbling notes.

"And when mothers eat selenium-rich ocean fish?"

He answered without hesitation.

"Improved neurological outcomes. Repeatedly."

She looked around the room, as though hoping others would meet her enthusiasm.

Some did.

Most didn't.

This was a room trained to wait for unanimity.

The chair closed her binder.

"We have to consider the political implications," she said. "If we revise the advisory, some will accuse us of bending to industry."

Nick lifted his gaze.

"Truth," he said quietly, "is not an industry."

A long silence settled over the room.

Committee members shifted in their seats — a few with discomfort, a few with relief, all of them newly aware that the vocabulary of fear no longer belonged exclusively to the past.

The chair spoke again, this time with a note of something that resembled humility.

"Your work suggests that the harm we feared is not the harm that exists."

He nodded once.

"We feared the wrong thing," he said.

"And now?" she asked.

"Now," he said, "we correct for that fear."

The room exhaled.

Not in agreement.

Not in surrender.

But in the soft, unmistakable way that institutions exhale when they finally sense the inevitability of change.

After the meeting, a subcommittee member caught up with him in the hallway.

She spoke in a low voice, as though stepping outside the formal weight of her position.

"Do you realize," she said, "that you're asking us to overturn a paradigm that has shaped two generations of clinicians?"

He didn't flinch.

"I'm asking you to honor the science," he said.

She shook her head — not in refusal, but in a quiet reckoning.

"It's just... so much to rewrite."

Nick looked at her gently.

"It's not rewriting," he said.

"It's finishing the sentence."

She inhaled sharply, as though something in her had shifted.

That evening, he walked back toward the river.

The sky had thinned into a pale dusk, the kind of light that makes the world look both larger and quieter. The river moved in long, deliberate sheets of softened ice, flowing with a certainty that no committee could replicate.

He leaned over the railing and watched the slow procession of ice.

Each fragment carried the same message:

The world resists correction

until correction becomes the only stable position.

He closed his eyes briefly, letting the cold air settle against his face.

He was not waiting for institutions to change.

He was walking through the season in which they finally could.

There were global bodies — the kind that issue declarations rather than guidelines — whose decisions shaped entire hemispheres of behavior. They met rarely, moved cautiously, and spoke in phrases polished by committees of committees. Nick had always regarded them with a mixture of respect and anthropological curiosity.

Today's session was one of those rare gatherings.

A multinational council had invited him to present—an assemblage of public health authorities, environmental ministers, nutrition advisors, ocean scientists, and policy delegates from fifteen countries. The meeting took place in a circular chamber designed to symbolize equality, though everyone in the room understood that influence tilted along predictable lines.

He took his seat near the perimeter, as he preferred. The center was for performance. The edges were for thinking.

The chair opened the session by reading a summary of the council's current stance on mercury in fish — a stance written in the language of a past decade: cautious, imprecise, shaped more by uncertainty than by evidence.

Nick listened with quiet patience.

When the chair finished, she turned to him.

"Dr. Ralston," she said, "we are revisiting our seafood advisories. Your work challenges long-held assumptions. We ask that you present your findings with full clarity."

He nodded and stepped forward.

He didn't speak immediately. He allowed the room to settle, to inhale, to prepare for the recalibration it didn't yet know it was about to undergo.

Then he began.

"Mercury," he said, "has dominated the conversation for fifty years."

The delegates watched him intently.

"But mercury," he continued, "is not the central variable. Selenium is."

This landed differently here — not with tension, not with skepticism, but with a kind of diplomatic surprise. People leaned back slightly, as if giving the idea room to expand.

He clicked to his first slide.

A global map.

Selenium levels in ocean fish across major fisheries.

"These data," he said, "are not recent. They are simply newly understood."

A delegate from northern Europe raised a hand.

"But we've built campaigns telling women to avoid fish," she said. "Are you saying the campaigns were wrong?"

He chose his words with care.

"I'm saying they were incomplete," he said. "And an incomplete truth becomes a distortion over time."

A delegate from South America spoke next.

"Our populations rely heavily on fish for nutrition," he said. "The warnings have caused real harm — people avoiding essential nutrients."

Nick nodded.

"Fear has a cost," he said. "And the cost compounds when the fear outlasts the evidence."

A senior official from East Asia leaned forward.

"If selenium is the protective factor," he said, "should our advisories emphasize consumption rather than avoidance?"

The entire room shifted — a literal, physical shift — as if the old frame had finally cracked just enough to let new air in.

"Yes," Nick said.

"One cannot avoid harm by avoiding nutrition. One avoids harm by understanding the interaction."

He let the sentence rest in the chamber.

Not pushed.

Not defended.

Simply placed.

During the break, a delegate approached him — a woman from a country where fish consumption was not just dietary but cultural.

She spoke quietly.

"I have spent ten years advising mothers to limit seafood," she said. "Your research suggests I have deprived them."

He shook his head gently.

"You protected them," he said. "But now you can nourish them."

Her eyes brightened — not with relief, but with recognition.

"And the world?" she asked.

"It will adjust," he said. "Slowly. But it will."

When the council reconvened, the chair asked him the question that had hovered unspoken for years.

"If we adopt your model," she said, "how long until the general public understands it?"

He looked around the room — at the flags, the nameplates, the delegates who had spent their careers balancing caution and clarity.

"The public," he said softly, "understands sooner than institutions think. They only need permission to update their understanding."

A diplomat from the Mediterranean added, "But what of the older advisories?"

"They remain part of the record," Nick said. "But records are not endpoints. They are waypoints."

The room fell into a reflective hush.

This was the moment — the hinge between decades of fear and decades of correction. No vote was taken. No declaration was issued. But the shift was unmistakable.

A paradigm had loosened.

Not collapsed.

Not replaced.

Loosened.

Enough to move.

When the session ended, he stepped outside into the evening air. The city lights shimmered across the water, and a slow breeze carried the scent of the harbor — briny, metallic, ancient.

He walked toward the shoreline.

The tide was moving in a quiet, deliberate rhythm — the kind of rhythm that had shaped continents long before human institutions tried to regulate fear.

He watched it for a long time.

The tide didn't care who agreed with it.

The tide didn't wait for consensus.

The tide didn't pause for committees.

The tide simply moved, as truth does.

Slow.

Steady.

Certain.

The world, he knew, was finally beginning to move with it.

There were scientific journals that behaved like fortresses — tall walls, narrow gates, guarded by reviewers whose caution was not unkind but immovable. These journals shaped the tone of entire disciplines. They acted as the memory of science, but also its delay.

Nick had learned to navigate them the way a seasoned mariner reads currents: not by force, not by argument, but by understanding the shape of resistance itself.

Today, one of those journals had summoned him for a closed-door review session — a rare event, used only when the implications of a manuscript extended beyond science into policy, economics, or public behavior.

The editorial board sat in a semicircle, each with a printed copy of his manuscript spread open before them. The margins were dense with handwritten notes — not corrections, but questions, hesitations, recalibrations.

He recognized that pattern instantly.

It meant they were close.

It meant they were afraid of being close.

The editor-in-chief spoke first.

"Dr. Ralston," she said, "your manuscript is strong. But we're concerned that its implications will be interpreted as a reversal of long-standing health guidance."

He nodded once.

“Implications,” he said, “are interpretations. My responsibility is the data.”

A senior reviewer leaned forward.

“But your data challenges the foundational narrative of mercury toxicity.”

“My data,” he said calmly, “completes it.”

Another reviewer — younger, sharper, with the look of someone who had built their career on molecular pathways — cleared his throat.

“The interaction model is elegant,” he said. “Beautiful, even. But beauty can be mistaken for persuasion.”

Nick met his gaze.

“Beauty,” he said softly, “is what science looks like when it stops resisting its own truth.”

The reviewer flushed — not embarrassed, but startled by the precision of the line.

The editor-in-chief tapped her pen against the table.

“Let’s address the core issue,” she said. “If we publish this, we signal that the paradigm has shifted.”

He didn’t speak for a long moment.

He allowed the silence to weigh itself.

Then, quietly:

“The paradigm shifted twenty years ago. The literature is only now approaching it.”

The board exchanged glances — the kind that reveal quiet, reluctant agreement.

One reviewer, a veteran in environmental health, finally asked:

"What is your goal here, Dr. Ralston? Be honest."

He answered with the simplicity of someone who had been carrying the truth long enough to know it didn't need embellishment.

"My goal," he said, "is accuracy. Nothing more. Nothing less."

"But accuracy disrupts," she said.

"Yes," he replied. "Accuracy always disrupts."

A deeper stillness fell across the room.

It was the sound of an institution realizing it had been living in a vocabulary that no longer fit the evidence.

After the formal questioning, a junior editor walked with him into the hallway. She held his manuscript against her chest the way a student holds a book that has unsettled them.

"May I ask something off-record?" she said.

He nodded.

"How do you stay patient?" she asked. "When the truth is obvious to you, but slow to everyone else?"

He studied her face — earnest, sincere, unguarded.

"Patience," he said, "is not waiting. Patience is knowing the truth doesn't need defending."

She blinked, caught off guard.

“And you really believe it will become consensus?”

He nodded gently.

“Consensus is inevitable,” he said. “Once the truth stops asking for permission.”

Later, he walked toward the far end of the campus, where the old greenhouse stood — a structure half-forgotten by new students but cherished by researchers who remembered what the university had once been. The glass panes were fogged from the sharp difference between interior humidity and the cold evening air.

He stepped inside.

The warmth enveloped him.

The scent of soil, chlorophyll, and old growth filled the space.

A row of plants stood under the soft glow of grow lights, their leaves trembling slightly in the imposed breeze of circulating fans.

This place always steadied him.

It reminded him that growth does not require agreement.

It requires conditions.

He walked slowly down the rows, touching nothing, observing everything. A graduate horticulture student looked up from her workbench and smiled awkwardly, surprised to see someone from the biochemical sciences wandering through her greenhouse.

"Sorry," she said. "I didn't expect anyone else tonight."

He returned the smile.

"Growth doesn't expect visitors," he said. "It simply continues."

She tilted her head, unsure whether she had heard something profound or simply literal.

He stepped back outside.

The cold hit him like a clarifying thought.

Above, the sky was a sheet of dim light — the kind of sky that sits between seasons, refusing to declare itself. The air smelled faintly of winter and faintly of thaw, as if undecided.

He walked toward the river.

Tonight, the river was quieter than usual.

The ice had thinned into long, glassy surfaces that drifted with an almost imperceptible glide.

They reflected the faint city glow, shimmering like fragments of an unfinished idea.

He stood there, hands in his pockets, observing the movement that required no audience.

The truth, he thought, moves like this.

Not fast.

Not dramatic.

But with absolute certainty.

Eventually, the world catches up.

There were seasons in a scientist's life when the work no longer belonged solely to the lab or the lecture hall — when it entered the bloodstream of an entire field, altering the way people thought even before they realized the shift had taken place. Nick had reached that season. It didn't feel triumphant. It felt... atmospheric. The way dawn feels just before the sun acknowledges it.

This time, the setting wasn't a conference, a committee, or a global chamber.

It was a classroom — the quietest place where revolutions begin.

He had agreed to guest-lecture for a cohort of graduate students whose advisor insisted they were "the most promising group in years." He arrived early, as he always did, and sat in the back of the room while they filed in, talking over each other in that kinetic, caffeinated rhythm unique to early scientists.

None of them carried the old fear.

None of them bowed to inherited anxieties.

They were unburdened, unscarred, unshaped by thirty years of mercury warnings.

They were, in effect, the future.

When he stepped to the podium, the room snapped into focus.

Not because he was famous.

Not because he was a myth.

But because they had read him — truly read him — in journals, in lectures, in citations buried inside hundred-page theses.

To them, he wasn't controversial.

He was foundational.

That alone was its own quiet victory.

He began without slides.

"I want to ask a question," he said. "And I want you to answer honestly."

The students straightened.

"What is the function of selenium in neurodevelopment?"

Hands shot up immediately.

A young man in the front row answered first.

"Selenoenzymes manage oxidative stress and support neural protection."

A woman added, "They're required for structural integrity in fetal brain development."

Another chimed in, "Deficiency predicts neurodevelopmental deficits regardless of mercury levels."

Nick nodded.

Every answer was correct.

He let the room breathe for a moment.

“Now,” he said, “what is the primary biochemical risk of mercury exposure?”

Silence.

Then a single voice:

“It binds selenium.”

“And by binding selenium...” he prompted.

“It disrupts the enzymes,” another said.

“And without those enzymes?”

“The brain loses protection.”

He smiled faintly.

“Good,” he said. “Now tell me why the public still thinks mercury is the problem.”

The room shifted — not from ignorance, but from discomfort.

They knew the answer.

They just didn’t like saying it.

Finally, one student spoke:

“Because fear was easier to communicate.”

A quiet murmur moved through the room — recognition, alignment, completion.

“Yes,” he said.

“And because fear arrived first.”

They absorbed that with the seriousness it deserved.

Then he asked the real question — the one that bridged generations.

"How long does it take," he said, "for a scientific truth to outlive its fear?"

A young woman in the back raised her hand.

"A generation," she said.

He shook his head gently.

"No," he said. "It takes two."

A murmur of surprise.

"Why two?" another asked.

"Because the first generation unlearns," he said.

"And the second generation no longer remembers what needed unlearning."

The students wrote that down — all of them — though the idea wasn't meant to be written. It was meant to be carried.

After the lecture, several lingered around him as students do when they sense they've been allowed to witness the turning of a page.

One asked, "Do you think our generation will shift the paradigm completely?"

He looked at them — the open faces, the unburdened posture, the absence of inherited fear — and something inside him softened.

"You already have," he said.

Another student approached hesitantly.

"I grew up being told fish was dangerous," she said quietly. "My mom avoided it during her pregnancy with my sister. But learning your work... it feels like a betrayal of what we were taught. And a relief. Both."

He nodded gently.

"That's how truth feels," he said. "When it arrives late."

She blinked, visibly moved.

"How did you keep going?" she asked.

He considered that for a long moment.

Then, simply:

"I didn't expect the world to agree with me," he said. "I expected the science to agree with itself. That was enough."

One of the students whispered to another, "That's actually beautiful."

Nick pretended he hadn't heard.

When he left the building, the campus was wrapped in a pale wash of winter light — the kind that dissolves edges and makes everything appear suspended, waiting.

He began his familiar walk toward the river, the footsteps steady, unhurried, shaped by decades of repetition.

The river had shifted again.

The ice was now thin, ribboned, translucent — moving with a certainty that required no stability and no permission.

He leaned on the railing.

Today, the river didn't look like correction.

It looked like inheritance — the world passing something forward, quietly, without ceremony.

He watched the long sheet of ice curve around a bend, as if performing the same gesture he had been making his entire career:

Clarity that moves

whether or not anyone notices

when it begins.

There were moments — rare, unplanned, unannounced — when the work revealed its true weight not through resistance or debate, but through recognition that arrived from unexpected directions. Nick never chased these moments. He didn't need to. They tended to find him precisely because he had never asked for them.

This one appeared in the quietest possible setting:

a small office tucked away in an administrative wing of the university, where the walls were lined with grant folders, student records, and the soft exhaustion of people who keep institutions running without ever being photographed for brochures.

He had been called in by an associate dean — a woman known for her precision, her skepticism, and her ability to see both the scientific and political implications of research. She wasn't easily impressed. She wasn't easily persuaded. She lived in the space between endorsement and caution.

When he stepped into her office, she closed the door with a deliberateness that hinted at the seriousness of what she wanted to say.

“Thank you for making the time,” she said. “I wanted to speak privately.”

He waited.

No assumptions.

No anticipation.

She sat down across from him and folded her hands on the desk.

“I attended your graduate seminar last week,” she said. “I didn’t announce myself. I wanted to hear how students interpret your work without you guiding them.”

He nodded.

“And?” he asked gently.

She exhaled.

“Your framework isn’t controversial to them,” she said. “It’s obvious.”

He didn’t smile, didn’t react. He simply absorbed it the way a person absorbs weather — quietly, respectfully, without claiming credit for it.

She continued.

"Their questions weren't defensive. They weren't protective of the old paradigm. They spoke of selenium, mercury interaction, enzyme protection, neural development... as if the integration had already happened."

"It has," he said.

"But it hasn't happened institutionally," she countered. "It hasn't happened globally. It hasn't even happened across all departments here."

He nodded again.

"Students," he said, "often arrive earlier than institutions."

She leaned back in her chair, studying him with a gaze that carried not admiration but something deeper — something like recalibration.

"You've been doing this for twenty-five years," she said. "I don't know how you stayed this patient."

He paused.

"When science is patient," he said, "the scientist learns to be."

She let that line settle, and for a long moment, the room felt completely still.

Then she leaned forward again.

"I want to propose something," she said. "A shift in the way our university presents seafood nutrition to incoming medical students. A revision of the materials. A reframing of the biochemical model."

This was a moment many scientists would have greeted with visible excitement.

He didn't.

Not out of indifference — but because the moment wasn't about him.

"What kind of reframing?" he asked.

"A truthful one," she said. "Not cautious. Not euphemistic. Just... correct."

He studied her expression.

Correction.

Not "update."

Not "adjustment."

Correction.

Finally.

"What changed your mind?" he asked.

She looked down at her desk, then at him — eyes steady, earnest.

"I realized," she said, "that the only thing keeping the old paradigm alive is our fear of admitting it's old."

He blinked.

Not in surprise.

In recognition.

"And?" he prompted.

"And I'm tired of protecting fear," she said. "I want to protect accuracy."

A subtle shift — barely perceptible — passed through him.

A quiet softening behind the eyes.

Not triumph.

Not relief.

Alignment.

"That can be done," he said.

She nodded.

"We'll take it slowly," she said. "But not quietly."

He stood, thanked her, and stepped back into the hallway.

The door clicked shut behind him.

He walked not toward his office, not toward the lab — but toward the long corridor leading to the river path. He didn't need fresh air. He needed proportion.

Outside, the day held that faint metallic brightness of late winter, when the sun is present but not yet warm. The river had evolved again — not dramatically, but distinctly. The ice was now a constellation of small, drifting fragments that caught the light like scattered glass.

He stopped at the railing.

Today, the river did not resemble correction.

It did not resemble thaw.

It resembled agreement — the quiet moment when an entire landscape acknowledges a change without announcing it.

He watched one piece of ice dip beneath another, merge, separate, glide.

Nothing dramatic.

Everything inevitable.

His work had never been about proving.

It had always been about aligning.

And now, at last, alignment had begun to arrive from places that had once resisted it — not out of pressure, but out of recognition.

The kind of recognition that stays.

He watched the slow procession of ice until the cold settled through his coat and into his bones in that steady, grounding way he had always loved.

Then he turned back toward the campus.

The world, he knew, was finally starting to behave like the science.

There were evenings — quiet, unceremonial, unnoticed by anyone but him — when the work revealed something even deeper than progress. Not acceptance. Not recognition. Something subtler:

Reversal.

Not the dramatic kind, not a public mea culpa or institutional announcement, but the quiet reversal that happens when people who once resisted him begin using his language as if it had always been theirs.

It happened tonight, in an unexpected place:

a small scientific roundtable hosted by a neighboring department.

The topic was “Maternal Neurodevelopment: Current Gaps and Emerging Models.”

He had not been invited as a speaker — only as an observer.

Perfect. He preferred it that way.

He took a seat near the wall. A modest position. A vantage point.

Around the table sat seven faculty members — a mixture of senior researchers, mid-career clinicians, and two rising stars whose reputations had started to extend beyond the region. Coffee cups. Laptops. The low hum of a building settling into evening.

The discussion began with familiar cautions:

“Maternal exposure remains a concern...”

“We still need to communicate risk clearly...”

“The existing paradigm continues to shape public perception...”

No surprises.

But then something shifted.

A mid-career clinician — one who had once publicly dismissed his work on the basis of "insufficient consensus" — cleared her throat and said:

"We should revisit the selenium interaction."

The room paused.

Someone blinked.

Someone else froze mid-sip.

She continued.

"I've been reviewing the selenoenzyme pathways. Mercury's inhibition is dose-dependent, but the protective functions are selenium-dependent. We may have emphasized the wrong axis."

Another faculty member chimed in:

"Yes — exactly. The issue isn't mercury presence, it's selenium displacement."

A third added:

"And fetal neurodevelopment relies heavily on those enzymes. A selenium-rich diet, particularly through ocean fish, actually supports the brain."

He sat perfectly still.

They were quoting his work — his terms, his framing, his biochemical architecture — but as if they had discovered it themselves.

He didn't mind.

In fact, he preferred it.

Truth makes its greatest leap forward when people forget where it came from.

One of the younger researchers opened a slide on her laptop.

“We should build the new curriculum around the interaction model,” she said. “Students are already asking about it.”

Another nodded enthusiastically.

“Agreed. The old fish-avoidance narrative is outdated. We need to emphasize nutrient sufficiency, not fear.”

He didn’t speak.

Not yet.

He watched as the conversation expanded, evolved, aligned.

“For example,” one said, “the public conflates mercury exposure with harm. But it’s really selenium deficiency that increases vulnerability.”

“Exactly,” another added. “We need to teach that seafood isn’t the risk — it’s the solution.”

The oldest member of the group — a scholar known for his cautious rhetoric — quietly closed his binder.

“We’ve spent decades warning against something that wasn’t the threat,” he said. “Perhaps it’s time to correct the record.”

The word hung in the room.

Correct.

Not revise.

Not update.

Correct.

He finally leaned forward.

The group turned to him instantly — respectful, attentive, aware.

“I’m glad you’re moving in this direction,” he said softly. “The truth has been waiting for you.”

They absorbed that — not defensively, not embarrassed — but with the quiet relief of people who finally recognized the shape of what had been in front of them all along.

The senior scholar nodded.

“You were right early,” he said. “That’s always difficult.”

Nick offered a faint smile.

“Correction arrives when it’s ready,” he said. “Not when we are.”

They nodded again — a shared understanding settling across the table.

The kind that signals a paradigm is no longer shifting.

It has shifted.

He walked back across campus as dusk deepened into a soft, mottled blue. The lights in the science buildings glowed through tall windows. Shadows of students moved between benches and whiteboards. The hum of learning drifted into the cold air like a low chorus.

He took his familiar path toward the river.

Tonight, the river had transformed again.

The ice was almost gone — reduced to thin, drifting shards, scattered across a wide, dark surface that moved with a slow, confident current. The river no longer looked like correction or even alignment.

Tonight, it looked like continuation — the part of the process where the world begins carrying the truth forward without asking where it came from.

He leaned on the railing.

This was the moment he had never expected to witness:

the generation that once resisted him

now parroting the framework they used to fear,

the new generation inheriting the corrected model

as though it had always been the model,

and the science behaving exactly as nature behaves:

slow,

steady,

inevitable,

indifferent to old narratives,

loyal only to truth.

A thin ribbon of ice moved past him, glinting faintly in the last light of evening.

He watched it slip beneath the surface and disappear.

Not a symbol.

Not a metaphor.

A reminder.

Truth doesn't need to dominate a landscape.

It only needs to move through it.

There were dinners — modest, local, off-campus — where the most important conversations in a scientist's life unfolded not in formal language but in the unguarded honesty that appears only when people believe no one will record their words.

Tonight was one of those dinners.

A small place near the edge of town, quiet enough that conversations didn't have to compete with anything but the soft clatter of dishes. The lighting was low. The tables were close. The kind of establishment where visiting scholars often ended up after long symposium days, wanting something real after hours of abstraction.

Nick had been invited by two senior colleagues and a younger researcher who insisted she needed "perspective." They chose a table near the window. Outside, the streetlights glowed in a soft halo of cold air, casting a pale shimmer on the thin snow along the sidewalk.

Menus folded shut.

Coats draped over the backs of chairs.

A pot of tea arrived.

And then, as often happened around him, the real conversation began.

It started innocently, with the younger researcher asking, “Do you ever feel like the field was stuck because we were afraid of the wrong thing?”

He looked at her for a long moment — not surprised by the question, but by how cleanly she had articulated it.

“Yes,” he said. “For a very long time.”

One of the senior scholars added, “Fear has a way of becoming architecture when it lasts long enough.”

Nick nodded.

“And architecture,” he said, “is hard to renovate.”

The younger researcher leaned forward.

“But what created the fear? The data never fully supported the mercury panic.”

The senior scholar responded, “The panic wasn’t scientific. It was cultural. People fear what they can name. Mercury was easy to name.”

“And selenium?” she asked.

The table fell quiet.

Nick finally answered.

"Selenium was harder to explain," he said. "And harder to fear. It doesn't behave like a villain. It behaves like a guardian."

The younger researcher smiled faintly.

"Guardians don't make headlines."

"No," he said. "But they make healthy children."

The table absorbed that.

Then one of the senior colleagues — the kind of man whose career spanned eras — set down his teacup and said something Nick had never expected to hear so openly.

"We were unfair to you."

Nick didn't respond.

Not out of discomfort — out of respect.

The man continued.

"You were ahead of the field. We weren't ready. And instead of admitting that, we questioned your timing."

Nick exhaled softly — not in relief, not in vindication, but in that quiet way a person breathes when someone finally names something he had carried alone for years.

He didn't look triumphant.

He didn't need to.

He simply said:

"Science isn't a race. It's a sequence. Some truths arrive early. Recognition arrives late."

The other senior scholar leaned back in his chair.

“Still,” she said, “you held the line. Even when people misunderstood your work. Even when they misrepresented it.”

He shook his head gently.

“They weren’t misrepresenting me,” he said. “They were defending the framework that shaped them. People don’t resist the truth. They resist losing the version of themselves built around the old truth.”

The younger researcher whispered, “That’s... painfully accurate.”

The meal arrived.

Plates set down quietly.

Steam rising into the low light.

No one spoke for a while.

Not out of tension, but because the conversation had reached a level of honesty that takes a moment to settle into the room.

Finally, one of the senior scholars asked:

“Does it bother you? That your work will be absorbed into the consensus without your name attached to the shift?”

He shook his head.

“The work outlives the worker,” he said. “Recognition is a distraction. Accuracy is the goal.”

The younger researcher blinked hard — not emotional, but moved.

“So this is what integrity looks like,” she said quietly.

He smiled — a faint, almost apologetic smile.

“No,” he said. “This is what clarity looks like.”

When the dinner ended, he walked out into the cold night. The air was sharp, clean, crystalline. The snow on the ground glowed faintly under the streetlights.

He didn’t walk back toward campus.

Not yet.

Instead, he turned toward the river.

He reached the familiar railing and stood silently, listening.

Tonight, the river made a different sound — not the brittle rush of thawing ice, not the soft brushing of drifting sheets, but a deeper, smoother movement. The surface was nearly clear now, the last fragments of ice gliding without resistance.

The river was no longer in transition.

It had entered its next state.

It didn’t announce the change.

It didn’t celebrate it.

It simply moved forward.

He watched the water slip past, dark and sure, carrying reflections of distant lights in long, unbroken lines.

The truth, he realized, had begun doing the same.

It no longer needed him to push it.

It no longer needed him to defend it.

It was gliding now — carried by the very people who once doubted it.

That was the moment he had earned, not through victory, but through persistence.

He rested his hands on the cold railing and let the quiet surround him.

The river had become the model.

And the world had finally begun following its current.

There were interviews — the quiet, recorded kind that were archived more than broadcast — where a scientist's words became part of the historical record whether he intended them to or not. Nick had given hundreds of interviews in his career, but this one felt different the moment he sat down.

It wasn't the setting.

Just a small media room in the communications wing.

Soft lights.

A plain table.

Two microphones.

A camera with a blinking red light.

What made it different was the interviewer.

A young journalist, not yet jaded, not yet shaped by the hardened angles of national media. She asked questions the way scientists analyze specimens — carefully, respectfully, without assuming she already understood the answer.

She began in a way no one else ever did.

“Dr. Ralston,” she said, “I don’t want to ask about mercury. I want to ask about time. Why does truth take so long to land?”

He folded his hands, considering her.

Most interviewers wanted conflict.

Most wanted drama.

Most wanted him to say something sharp about the agencies that resisted him.

She wanted something else.

“It takes long,” he said, “because people confuse the first model they learn with the final model that exists.”

She nodded slowly.

“So the problem isn’t the science,” she said, “it’s the loyalty to the first story.”

He smiled faintly.

“Yes,” he said. “And the more dramatic the first story, the harder it is to replace.”

She leaned forward.

“Do you think your work arrived too early?”

He paused before answering.

"No," he said. "The science arrived when it needed to. The understanding arrived when it could."

The journalist blinked, visibly struck by that distinction.

"So you never wanted to be first?" she asked.

"I wanted to be accurate," he said. "Accuracy ages well. Urgency does not."

She exhaled — like someone hearing something she wished she'd heard in school.

She consulted her notes.

"I've read papers from the early 2000s," she said. "Your interaction model was there — fully formed, fully argued. But it didn't change policy. Why?"

He didn't flinch.

"Because policy responds to consensus, not clarity."

"Is that a flaw?" she asked.

"It's a limitation," he said. "But not a flaw. Consensus protects the public from reckless revision. It also slows necessary correction. The challenge is knowing when the slowdown becomes harmful."

"And with seafood advisories?" she pressed.

"We reached that point," he said.

The journalist looked down, then back up.

"One more question," she said quietly. "Do you ever feel bitter?"

He could have given the easy answer.

He could have said no.

He could have said the work was its own reward.

Instead, he gave the correct answer.

"Bitterness comes from expecting recognition," he said. "I didn't expect recognition. I expected the truth to win. It's winning. That's enough."

She sat back, stunned by the tone — not triumphant, not defiant, simply grounded.

Then she asked the question that would live longest in the recording.

"What do you want the world to understand about what you've done?"

He didn't look at the camera.

He didn't straighten his posture.

He didn't rehearse a statement.

He just said:

"That I didn't change the science. I listened to it."

Silence.

Not empty silence.

Deep silence.

The kind that follows a sentence that cannot be improved.

The interviewer slowly stopped the recording.

"Thank you," she said softly. "Truly."

He nodded, gathered his notes, and left the room as quietly as he had entered it.

Outside, evening had settled into a soft slate-blue light. A light that dissolved edges, made distances indistinct, and turned the campus into a study in gradients.

He walked the familiar path toward the river.

Tonight, the river was fully free — glass-dark, fluid, carrying no memory of the ice that had once encased it. The current moved with long, unbroken lines of motion that gave the surface the appearance of thought rather than water.

He stood at the railing.

There was no metaphor left to impose on the river.

It had surpassed metaphor.

Tonight, the river simply was — moving forward, not in defiance of the season behind it, but because the season behind it had completed its work.

That, he realized, was the shape of his career.

He didn't replace the old model.

He completed it.

He didn't defeat the old warnings.

He outlived them.

He didn't correct the science.

He clarified it.

And now the current was carrying the truth, with or without him, exactly as it should.

He closed his eyes—not to rest, but to listen.

The water had no applause to give.

Only continuity.

And continuity was enough.

There were annual reports — those dense, glossy documents that institutions publish more for themselves than for the public — where language is chosen not for accuracy but for political survivability. Nick rarely paid attention to them. They were artifacts of administrative life, not scientific life.

But this year, something unusual happened.

A colleague slipped a draft of the university's upcoming research report under his office door. No note. No explanation. Just a quiet gesture that said, You might want to see this.

He didn't open it immediately.

He set it on the corner of his desk, where it sat like an unopened letter that carries a pulse.

Only after he finished responding to a student's email, only after he cleaned up a spreadsheet of enzyme data, only after he poured a cup of coffee — only then did he sit down and open the glossy draft.

He turned the pages slowly.

- A feature on climate modeling.
- A highlight of aerospace engineering.
- A spread on rural health disparities.
- A piece on grain genetics.

He moved through them without attachment.

Then he reached the page titled "Emerging Paradigms in Maternal Nutrition."

He stopped.

There, in clean university language — cautious but undeniably precise — was the framework he had carried for twenty-five years:

"Recent advancements emphasize the critical protective role of selenium in fetal neurodevelopment and its interaction with mercury exposure. Current evidence suggests that nutritional sufficiency, rather than avoidance, may represent a more accurate model for promoting healthy outcomes."

He blinked.

Not dramatically.

Just once.

A single blink that acknowledged:

This is new.

He kept reading:

“Ongoing work by university researchers has contributed significantly to this reframing, prompting updates to curricular materials and informing regional public health discussions.”

It didn’t name him.

It didn’t need to.

The language was his.

The architecture was his.

The shift was unmistakable.

This was how scientific revolutions appear in institutional writing:

first as rumor,

then as resistance,

then — if they survive long enough — as formal prose.

He leaned back in his chair.

He wasn’t moved by pride.

He was moved by proportion.

For the first time, the institution had mirrored the truth without flinching.

He closed the report and set it aside, knowing exactly what this meant:

The paradigm was no longer being discussed.

It was being absorbed.

Later that afternoon, he walked to the student union to pick up a cup of tea. He rarely came here — too noisy, too energetic, too filled with academic adolescence. But something about the day called him toward the atmosphere of those still learning.

Inside, the place buzzed with conversation and the low thrum of espresso machines.

He waited in line, quiet, unnoticed.

Ahead of him, two undergraduates — clearly in the biomedical track — were discussing a study guide one of them had annotated.

"I thought mercury was the main risk," one said, flipping pages.

"No," the other corrected. "It's selenium deficiency. If the enzymes don't have enough selenium, mercury causes problems. But if selenium is sufficient, fish is actually protective."

He stiffened imperceptibly.

The first student frowned. "Where'd you get that?"

"From Dr. Patel's lecture last week," the second said. "She changed her slides. Said it's the updated model."

Updated model.

Not controversial model.

Not emerging model.

Updated.

He didn't turn.

He didn't insert himself.

He didn't breathe differently.

He simply listened.

The first student said, "Huh. Makes sense when you say it like that."

And then — with the casual indifference of someone who has no idea they are participating in the correction of a generation — she added:

"I don't know why they didn't just teach us that from the beginning."

He felt something inside him soften — a quiet recognition that bordered on the transcendent.

There it was.

The moment every scientist works for but rarely gets to witness:

The new truth had become the assumed truth.

The next generation wasn't resisting the correction.

They were confused it had ever needed correcting.

He stepped aside, letting them order their drinks, then walked to the exit with his tea in hand.

He didn't smile.

He didn't need to.

The air outside was crisp, the sky a pale winter blue.

The walk toward the river felt lighter today, not because the burden had lifted, but because the burden had redistributed itself across a generation.

When he reached the river, he found a new surface waiting for him.

The ice was gone.

Completely gone.

The water flowed in a dark, uninterrupted ribbon — swift, certain, unbroken.

The river was not “free.”

The river was not “corrected.”

The river was not “transformed.”

The river was simply true — behaving exactly as a river behaves when its season aligns with its nature.

And that, he realized, was the state of his work.

It was no longer being corrected.

It was no longer pushing.

It was no longer resisting resistance.

It was flowing.

Forward.

Unbroken.

Unapologetic.

Unafraid.

He rested his hands on the cold railing.

Truth, once carried long enough, begins to carry itself.

There were international workshops — not the formal, agenda-driven summits of policymakers, but the liminal gatherings where researchers, clinicians, field workers, and nutrition specialists from around the world sat shoulder to shoulder in utilitarian chairs, sharing data in the raw, unpolished form where truth is easiest to see.

This one took place in a converted research hall attached to an institute overlooking a wide estuary. The windows were tall. The air smelled faintly of salt and metal. The room hummed with that polite chaos unique to multinational science: whispered translations, rustling papers, occasional laughter from people who had been arguing about biochemical pathways for decades.

Nick didn't present today.

He didn't need to.

His work was already in the room.

He sat near the side, listening.

A marine biologist from New Zealand was explaining their new findings on selenium-rich pelagic species. A Brazilian pediatrician was describing improved developmental outcomes in coastal communities after dietary shifts. A Scandinavian toxicologist was reviewing a recent longitudinal study that complicated long-held beliefs about mercury risk.

Nothing they said was new to him.

Everything they said was new to each other.

He watched quietly as the conversation began to cohere — the way threads come together long before the people holding them realize they are weaving the same fabric.

Then something happened.

A researcher from Japan — a respected figure, meticulous, cautious — stood and said:

“We have been focusing on mercury for too long. The evidence is clear that selenium availability determines vulnerability. The paradigm needs to shift from fear to balance.”

The room stilled.

People turned toward him.

She continued, unfazed.

“Our data supports the interaction model.”

A pause.

“The same model Dr. Ralston proposed more than two decades ago.”

A ripple moved through the room — not shock, not debate, but an almost physical recalibration. As if the space itself had adjusted to accommodate something that had, until this moment, been acknowledged only in fragments.

Someone else spoke up — a clinician from South Korea:

“Yes. And the new enzyme protection studies confirm his early work.”

A French researcher added, “We teach the interaction model now. Students find it intuitive.”

From the back, a Canadian epidemiologist said, “We are revising our national guidance to incorporate selenium sufficiency.”

And then the most unexpected voice joined:

A researcher from a country whose agencies had once resisted him most fiercely.

“Our ministry,” he said, “is reconsidering the advisories. We will likely adopt the interaction framework.”

A silence followed — not awkward, not tense, but historical.

Everyone in the room knew it.

It was the moment a paradigm ceased being “emergent” and became “established.”

Nick didn’t move.

Didn’t speak.

Didn’t shift in his chair.

But the air around him changed — subtly, undeniably — as though the entire room had rotated a few degrees toward the truth he’d been carrying all these years.

During the break, an older scientist approached him — someone who had once debated him publicly at a conference fifteen years earlier.

He extended a hand.

"I owe you an apology," he said.

Nick shook his head. "No you don't."

"Yes," the man insisted. "I resisted your findings because I was afraid of how much we'd have to rewrite. I wasn't protecting the science. I was protecting myself."

Nick studied him gently.

"You're protecting the science now," he said.

The man nodded with a mixture of humility and relief.

"I just wish I'd shifted sooner," he said.

"Everyone shifts when they can," Nick replied. "Not when we want them to."

Later in the afternoon, the workshop entered its final session: a roundtable on global harmonization of seafood advisories. The moderator asked for final comments from the room.

A young researcher — sharp, confident, unburdened by the old warnings — raised her hand.

"I think the guidance needs to reflect what we all now understand," she said. "That the primary risk to the fetus isn't mercury exposure. It is insufficient selenium.

We have to stop warning mothers away from the very food that protects their children."

Heads nodded around the room.

And then — without fanfare, without ceremony — one of the senior scientists said:

"Is anyone still defending the old model?"

Silence.

Not defensive silence.

Not stubborn silence.

A silence that meant:

No.

No one is.

The paradigm had tipped.

Not loudly.

Not publicly.

But definitively.

A shift twenty-five years in the making.

When the session ended, the researchers drifted out into the cold coastal air, their conversations trailing behind them like steam. Nick walked toward the estuary path, where the tide was high and moving with a dark, glassy certainty.

He stopped at the railing.

The water below was no longer broken by ice or slowed by winter.

It surged quietly, steadily, shaped only by the moon and its own underlying physics.

There was no metaphor left to impose.

The river had become the shape of the truth itself.

It moved because movement was its nature.

It aligned because the world had finally allowed it to.

It no longer needed correction.

It simply needed acknowledgment.

As he stood there, the tide shifted — a subtle, steady pulse that the body feels before the mind registers.

He closed his eyes.

For the first time in his career, the work felt lighter.

Not finished.

Never finished.

But carried.

Carried by others.

Carried by institutions.

Carried by the world.

And most importantly:

Carried by a generation that would never have to unlearn what the previous one had feared.

There were seasons in a scientist's life when the phone calls changed — not in frequency, not in urgency, but in tone. For two decades, most of Nick's calls had been requests for clarification, rebuttal, reassurance, or defense. People called him to confirm their doubts, to challenge his certainty, to question the timing of his conclusions.

But now the calls were different.

They were arriving from people who simply wanted to understand what they should have understood years ago.

People who were stepping into the correction rather than away from it.

This was one of those calls.

It came from a coastal physician — a respected clinician who had built her reputation around protecting pregnant mothers through strict seafood restrictions. She had enforced the old paradigm so fervently that her colleagues called her “the Mercury Sentinel.”

She had once challenged him on a panel, dismissing selenium’s protective role as “a theoretical footnote.”

Today, she called him directly.

Her voice was steady, but thin around the edges — the tone of someone who had begun confronting a truth she had previously rejected.

“Dr. Ralston,” she said. “I was reviewing my patient outcomes from the past twelve years. Something doesn’t add up.”

Nick didn’t move, didn’t speak, didn’t fill the space.

She continued.

"The mothers who avoided fish entirely... their children show more neurological deficits than the ones who ate ocean fish twice a week."

He waited.

Not to pressure her.

To let her arrive.

"I dismissed your model," she said quietly. "I never should have."

He responded with the calm that had shaped his entire career.

"You followed the guidance you were given," he said. "You protected your patients with the tools you had."

She inhaled sharply.

"But the tools were wrong," she said.

He didn't correct her. He didn't absolve her. He gave her the line she needed to step forward without collapsing under the weight of hindsight.

"The tools were incomplete," he said.

Silence — deep, receptive, painful silence.

Finally, she spoke again.

"I want to change the way I practice," she said. "But I don't know how to explain this shift to my patients."

He closed his eyes for a moment, letting the question settle into its own rightful depth.

"Explain it the way the science explains it," he said. "Tell them that the brain needs selenium. Tell them that fish provides it. Tell them that the warnings reflected what we knew then, and that our understanding has matured."

She exhaled, long and slow.

"Do you think they'll trust me?"

He answered gently.

"They'll trust your honesty."

A long pause — the kind in which someone reorders their professional identity.

"Thank you," she said finally. "For your patience. For your... persistence."

"Persistence," he said softly, "is simply listening to the truth longer than others can."

She ended the call, not with closure, but with continuity — the kind that signals the beginning of a new era in a single clinician's life.

He set the phone down and stepped outside.

Dusk was settling over campus, the sky washed in muted blues and grays. Students moved across walkways like small currents in a larger river. He walked slowly, without urgency, feeling the shape of the day in the crisp air.

The river drew him again.

He reached the familiar railing.

Tonight, the water moved with a new depth — darker, faster, almost luminous beneath the layered twilight. It no longer resembled transition, correction, thaw, alignment, or even continuation.

Tonight, it resembled succession — the moment when the old system hands its place to the new without ceremony, without announcement, without regret.

The river did not mourn the ice.

The ice had served its season.

The water did not rush to replace what had melted.

It simply took its place.

He watched a long, unbroken band of water slide under the bridge, carrying reflections that elongated and dissolved.

There was something profound in its movement:

truth replacing the space once held by fear,

accuracy overtaking the vacancy left by correction,

clarity inhabiting the room old warnings once occupied.

He rested his hand on the railing, feeling the cold metal anchor him.

He had expected resistance.

He had expected delay.

He had expected fatigue.

He had not expected this:

the world arriving at the truth

with the quiet dignity of a river reclaiming its channel.

He stood there for a long time.

Not proud.

Not relieved.

Not triumphant.

Aligned.

Ready.

Held by the continuity of a work that was no longer his burden alone.

There were post-conference evenings — the kind that did not end with applause or closing remarks, but with an almost electrical quiet that settles over a city when hundreds of minds have spent the day rearranging the architecture of a shared field. These were the evenings where breakthroughs did not announce themselves; they simply lingered in the corridors, in the walkways, in the space between departing conversations.

Nick found himself in one of those evenings now.

The symposium had ended hours ago. Attendees had dispersed to hotels, airports, restaurants, and train stations. The last shuttle had left. The courtyard lights had come on. The building had grown hollow with the peaceful emptiness that follows collective intellectual exhaustion.

He stayed behind.

Not because he needed solitude, but because he wanted to feel the afterimage of the day — the way a musician might remain in the hall after the audience leaves, listening to the last note vibrate in the rafters long after the instrument falls silent.

He stood inside the glass atrium, holding a conference program in one hand.

Page after page listed sessions that had once belonged to the fringe:

"Selenium Bioavailability and Fetal Outcomes"

"Rethinking Seafood Risk Communication"

"Neuroprotective Enzyme Interactions in Marine Diets"

"Maternal Nutrition: Updating the Global Model"

These were the conversations he used to have alone.

Now they were occupying rooms filled with people who had flown across oceans to hear them.

He slipped the program into his coat and walked out into the night.

The city smelled of cold stone and late autumn leaves. He followed a narrow street that led down to the waterfront, passing cafés lit by soft amber bulbs and restaurants where researchers were still arguing, still parsing their disagreements, still discovering points of unexpected consensus.

He crossed a pedestrian bridge, stopping at the center where the river widened into the bay.

The water below was restless — not turbulent, not loud, but insistent. A tide of thousands of small, overlapping currents. The surface looked like thought itself: continuous, layered, alive.

For the first time, the river did not feel like metaphor.

It felt like record.

A ledger of all the moments that had brought him here:

The early grants that went nowhere.

The colleagues who supported him quietly.

The ones who resisted publicly.

The mothers who emailed with confusion and fear.

The agencies that refused to update their advisories.

The long nights of recalculating data in an empty lab.

The slow recognition that clarity takes a generation, not a year.

And now, the unmistakable shift:

the field had begun referencing his work not as disruption, but as foundation.

He rested his elbows on the railing and looked out across the water.

The city lights traced broken ribbons across the surface — gold, blue, white — stretching, bending, dissolving as the tide moved. Their distortions didn't erase the reflection; they completed it.

He thought about the students who now learned the corrected model first.

About the clinicians who were rewriting their guidance.

About the researchers adjusting their frameworks.

About the policymakers beginning to reform advisories without waiting for permission.

He thought about the younger audiences — the ones who hear him speak in Europe, Asia, South America — who raise their hands not to challenge the premise, but to develop it.

They ask:

"How do we apply this in our fisheries?"

"What does this mean for early childhood policies?"

"When will the international guidelines update?"

"What comes next?"

What comes next.

That had always been the right question.

Because the truth wasn't the destination.

The truth was the baseline.

The floorboard on which the next generation would build something bigger than the correction itself.

He felt the night air settle around him, cool and steady.

Somewhere behind him, a public clock chimed the hour — not ceremonially, not significantly, just to mark time's simple progression.

He closed his eyes.

He did not feel the need to be vindicated.

He did not feel the need to be remembered.

He did not feel the need to be credited.

He felt something better:

continuity.

The knowledge that his work was entering the world's bloodstream, slow and permanent, like a nutrient that had been missing for too long.

He stood there a moment longer, listening to the water.

Then he opened his eyes.

And walked on.

There were university mornings — the kind that arrive not with urgency but with an understated authority, as though the institution itself is reminding everyone that knowledge, despite its politics and its delays, still advances by the steady discipline of showing up.

This morning was like that.

Nick crossed the quad at an hour when most students were still inside, the air carrying the faint metallic scent of late fall. The sidewalks were damp from a night rain, and the sky hovered in that pale vacancy between silver and blue.

He walked toward the building where he had lectured, researched, and mentored for years. Not because he had a class today — he didn't — but because something in him wanted to see the hallway that had become its own kind of chronicle.

That hallway had witnessed everything:

The first time he put up the early interaction diagrams.

The discouraging conversations with administrators.

The unexpected encouragements from visiting scholars.

The printed studies that contradicted the old paradigm.

The departmental debates — some polite, some not.

The slow migration of younger faculty toward his framework.

And now, the subtle but undeniable shift in tone.

He entered the building, letting the silence surround him.

The halls were lined with display cases containing academic posters from past symposia. Most portrayed fields with fast-moving consensus — engineering, materials science, aerospace. But tucked into the middle section were the nutrition and biochemical posters, their bright colors faded slightly under the fluorescent lights.

He walked until he reached the section devoted to maternal health.

And there it was.

A new poster.

Sleek.

Modern.

Minimal.

Not his work — the design style made that obvious.

But unmistakably built on his foundation.

“Selenium Biomarkers and Fetal Neuroprotection:

A Revised Framework for Clinical Practice.”

He leaned in.

The abstract articulated, without fanfare:

- the enzyme dependencies,
- the nutrient interactions,
- the hierarchy of vulnerabilities,
- the insufficiency of mercury-alone models,
- and the need to shift public guidance toward balance rather than avoidance.

And then the sentence that quietly rewrote twenty years of debate:

“Emerging evidence supports the model in which selenium sufficiency, rather than mercury avoidance, plays the primary role in protecting fetal neurodevelopment.”

He exhaled through his nose — not dramatically, but with a kind of grounded, internal recognition.

This was how paradigms finalize themselves.

Not through victories.

Through posters.

He stepped back and let the poster simply exist, taking its place in the hallway where undergraduates, graduate students, faculty, visiting researchers, and donors would pass it.

It struck him that the poster wasn't competing with anything around it.

There was no argument.

No counterpoint.

No dissenting model pinned up alongside it.

The correction had become normal.

He turned and continued walking until he reached the stairwell. He descended slowly, his hand gliding along the rail, each step echoing with a faint metallic resonance.

At the base of the stairs, he pushed open the door that led outside.

The river called to him again.

It was strange — he had walked this route so many times over the years, but now it felt less like habit and more like ritual, as though each pass was acknowledging a different stage of the work.

Today, the river was a muted steel-gray, thickened by the slow churn of seasonal transition. The banks were dark and soft, coated with the damp residue of early freeze. A thin mist rose from the water, dissolving as it reached the taller air.

He stood at the railing, letting the quiet settle.

The water moved with the deliberate cadence of something that had survived winter many times and refused to be hurried by spring. It carried a weight to it now — not burdensome, but dignified.

The truth he had carried for so long had taken the river's form:

neither rushed nor delayed,

neither announced nor hidden,

neither triumphant nor obscure.

Simply present.

Simply continuous.

Simply correct.

He could no longer remember the last time he felt the need to defend the model.

That itself was a sign — not of victory, but of succession.

A generation had taken hold.

An institution had recalibrated.

A field had matured.

A world had begun to reconsider.

He placed both hands on the railing, absorbing the cold through his palms.

The river, indifferent to acknowledgment, flowed on.

He watched it, unhurried.

The continuity was enough.

There were institutional conversations — the quiet, strategic ones that occur not in conference rooms or policy forums, but in offices where the blinds are half-drawn and the door is only mostly closed. This was one of those conversations.

It began with an email.

A short one.

“Could you stop by?”

No subject line.

No explanation.

Just a request from an administrator who had spent years balancing on the thin edge between scientific honesty and bureaucratic caution.

Nick went.

Not out of obligation, but out of curiosity.

When institutions change, they rarely announce it.

They whisper first.

He knocked gently and stepped inside.

The administrator — a woman who had once asked him, with genuine concern, whether his model was “too destabilizing for public messaging” — gestured toward a chair.

“I wanted your thoughts on something,” she said.

He nodded.

She slid a folder across the desk.

“Public Health Advisory Draft — Internal Review Only.”

He opened it.

The language was new.

Not radical.

Not bold.

But unmistakably shifted.

The draft no longer warned against seafood consumption during pregnancy.

It recommended ensuring adequate selenium intake first, then evaluating mercury exposure within that context.

A foundational rearrangement.

The kind that rewrites guidance without appearing to.

He read silently.

After a page and a half, he stopped.

“Who wrote this?” he asked.

“Working group,” she said.

Then, after a pause:

“But your work is in every paragraph.”

He looked back at the document.

“Do they know that?”

"They do," she said. "The question is whether the public will."

He closed the folder gently.

"The public will know what we tell them," he said. "If we tell them accurately, they will understand accurately. If we tell them partially, they will fear partially."

She folded her hands.

"And if we tell them differently from what we told them for twenty years?"

He met her eyes.

"Then we tell them the truth grew. That's what science does."

She nodded — slowly, with the expression of someone who had carried a set of assumptions for far too long and had begun to feel their weight.

"There's one more concern," she said.

He waited.

"Some members worry that updating the advisory implies we were wrong."

He shook his head gently.

"It implies we are learning."

She inhaled.

"That's not always how institutions like to frame things."

He smiled, but only in the way that someone does when they've lived the truth long enough to see its resistance soften.

"Institutions don't have to like it," he said. "They just have to allow it."

She sat back, absorbing that.

Then:

"We'd like your guidance as we finalize this."

His response was quiet, measured.

"Make the correction without apology.

Make the guidance without fear.

Make the messaging without drama.

The science is ready.

The world is nearly ready."

Her shoulders dropped slightly — not in defeat, but in relief.

"Thank you," she said.

He stood.

"Call me when the next draft is ready."

As he left the office, he didn't feel victorious.

He felt something deeper:

The institution had shifted from defending the past to preparing the future.

That was the fulcrum.

The turning of the axis.

Outside, the sky had changed.

Gray had surrendered to a deeper, richer blue.

The air held that quiet tension that precedes a winter sunset.

He walked steadily toward the river.

He wasn't thinking about policy anymore.

Or advisories.

Or recognition.

He was thinking about continuity.

The kind that extends beyond any single scientist's lifetime.

When he reached the water's edge, the river was moving with a strange, almost sculptural calm — wide, slow, but undeniably powerful. The surface held its own internal logic: not chaotic, not placid, but inevitable.

It resembled the final stage of a paradigm shift:

silent, steady, irreversible.

He rested his hands on the railing.

A gust of wind moved across the water, reshaping the reflections into long silver ribbons.

For a moment, he felt the scale of it — the decades, the resistance, the clarity, the slow alignment, the new generation rising into a model they would take for granted.

He closed his eyes.

There was no need to imagine the future.

It had already begun.

There were departures — not endings, not farewells, but the quieter kind of departures that happen when a field shifts beneath your feet and you realize the work you've spent a lifetime carrying has begun to walk forward without you.

It happened on a Thursday.

Nothing remarkable about the day.

Classes in session.

Lab windows fogged in the corners.

Students with backpacks moving in loose currents across the quad.

But there was a meeting.

A routine departmental meeting — the kind where agendas are discussed, curricula revised, budgets debated, and updates shared with the polite imprecision of academic life.

Nick sat toward the end of the long conference table, not out of strategy but habit. The younger faculty filled the front seats with the gentle ambition that accompanies early careers. Older faculty scattered themselves around the perimeter, their faces etched with a familiarity that had matured into a kind of academic seasonality.

The chair began with announcements.

New grants.

Seminar schedules.

Visiting scholars.

Accreditation updates.

Then came the curriculum revisions.

A younger professor — sharp, composed, earnest — stood to review changes to the undergraduate nutrition sequence.

"We've updated Module 3," she said, adjusting her glasses. "The section on seafood advisories now reflects the interaction model. We removed the old mercury-focused framing."

A few nods.

No resistance.

No debate.

No side conversations.

She continued:

"We've rewritten the fetal neurodevelopment lecture. It now centers on selenium-dependent enzymes and the protective interaction with dietary mercury. Students have responded well to the clarity."

Nick watched the room.

No one blinked.

No one hesitated.

No one took a defensive posture.

The new model had not been introduced.

It was now simply what the program teaches.

The chair nodded.

“Good. It’s time for the curriculum to reflect the science.”

Time.

As if it had just become time.

As if time had always been this gentle.

She went on:

“We’re updating the exam bank too — removing questions that assume mercury avoidance is the primary recommendation for pregnant women.”

Another nod from the room.

It was done.

No ceremony.

No acknowledgement.

No attribution.

The model he carried for twenty-five years had been fully embedded into the institution’s teaching structure.

And in that moment, something subtle happened inside him — not pride, not relief, but a kind of release.

The work was no longer his.

It belonged to the next generation.

He had been the origin point,

but they were now the continuity.

After the meeting, he walked out of the building alone.

The late afternoon sun cast long gold stripes across the pavement. Students hurried past him, laughing, oblivious to the quiet turning point that had just taken place in a small conference room on the second floor.

He crossed the quad, passing beneath the last of the autumn leaves — crisp, curled, holding the final light.

He walked toward the river.

It was becoming instinct now, the way some people return to a childhood street or a chapel. The river had become his measure, his mirror, his companion through the long correction.

When he reached the railing, the river was wide and calm — a slow, uncompromising movement beneath the cooling sky.

For a long moment, he didn't think about anything.

He just listened.

The water moved as it always had, unconcerned with who understood it, who resisted it, who ignored it, who fought it, who finally embraced its pattern.

The river didn't require consensus to be correct.

It only required time.

And now the science had caught up to the river's temperament — slow, precise, irreversible.

He exhaled softly, letting the breath dissolve into the cold air.

The world would continue the work.

The students would continue the work.

The institutions would continue the work.

The science, finally, would continue the work.

The river had always known this.

He rested his hands on the railing.

Continuity — full, mature, unburdened — carried the truth forward.

He watched the current for a long time.

There were recognitions — not awards, not ceremonies, not anything with a podium or a plaque, but the quieter recognitions that happen in a field when people begin to cite a scientist not for novelty or controversy, but for orientation. It is the point at which a body of work is no longer debated, no longer defended, no longer framed in opposition to something else. It is simply where the compass points.

This recognition came slowly, almost imperceptibly, and then all at once.

It began with an email from a doctoral student overseas — concise, polite, written with the precision of someone trained in a system that values order.

“Dr. Ralston, I hope you don’t mind me reaching out.

Our team is designing a longitudinal study on coastal maternal diets.

My advisor told me, ‘Begin with the interaction model.’

He meant your work.

Could we ask for your guidance?”

There was no fanfare in the message.

No attempt to flatter.

No retrospective apology for past misunderstandings.

Just an assumption:

Start where the truth already lives.

He wrote back with the same steady tone he used with all young scientists:

“Send me your design draft.

I’ll help you strengthen the enzyme metrics.”

He didn’t think much of it.

But a week later, another message arrived — this one from a research team in Chile studying selenium-rich coastal species.

Two days later, one from Iceland.

Then one from a medical school in Singapore.

Then a public health team in Kenya preparing new maternal nutrition guidelines.

All asking him the same quiet question:

"Can we align our work with yours?"

Not "debate," not "clarify," not "challenge."

Align.

He wasn't being consulted to defend the model anymore.

He was being consulted to extend it.

Then came the moment that confirmed, without any doubt, that the paradigm had not only shifted — it had settled.

A package arrived at his office.

Inside was a newly released global nutrition textbook — one of the most widely used in medical schools. He flipped to the maternal health chapter.

There it was.

The interaction model.

Not as a sidebar.

Not as an alternative theory.

Not as a late chapter footnote.

But as the framework.

The diagrams were new, the graphics modern, the colors bold — but the architecture was unmistakable. He traced a finger along the biochemical pathways he had once drawn by hand on whiteboards in cramped classrooms.

Then he read the caption beneath a key illustration:

“Neuroprotective enzyme systems depend primarily on selenium sufficiency.

Mercury’s potential effects must be evaluated through this lens.”

And then, the understated line:

“This model, now widely adopted, reflects the scientific consensus that has emerged over the past two decades.”

Consensus.

The word landed gently.

Not triumph.

Not validation.

Not victory.

Consensus.

It meant the science had absorbed the truth so thoroughly that it no longer required defense.

He closed the textbook softly, like someone handling an object that carried both weight and grace.

That afternoon, he walked slowly across campus. The air held the crisp neutrality of late-season weather —

neither the urgency of winter nor the promise of spring, but the in-between clarity where everything is seen for what it is.

He followed the familiar path toward the river.

The water today was almost impossibly smooth — a wide plane of muted silver, reflecting clouds that drifted like slow, contemplative thoughts. At the far end of the bend, a strip of darker water pulsed steadily, marking the deeper channel.

He leaned on the railing.

The river felt different now.

It had long ceased being metaphor.

Then it had become record.

Then it had become mirror.

Now it was something beyond all of those.

It had become continuation — the movement that persists regardless of who watches it, who measures it, who interprets it, who doubts it, who accepts it.

He realized then that the science had taken on the river's temperament:

- Unhurried.
- Undeniable.
- Self-correcting.
- Self-sustaining.

- Self-moving.

He closed his eyes.

For the first time since he began this work, he felt the world catching up not with him, but with the truth itself.

He had never expected to witness that in his lifetime.

He opened his eyes again, watching as a gust of wind brushed the water and carried a series of ripples diagonally across the surface.

The truth was no longer his to bear.

It was part of the current now.

Permanent.

Quiet.

Irreversible.

Carried.

He remained there, listening to the subtle rhythm of the river against the banks.

There were letters — the kind sent not for flattery, not for networking, not for academic positioning, but Because Someone Needed To Tell the Origin Story Right. They came from places with coastlines, places with river deltas, places with fisheries, places where mothers had been warned for a generation to fear the very food that would have protected their children.

These were not long letters.

They were not dramatic.

They did not describe transformation in grand terms.

But they carried weight.

One came from a public health nurse in Alaska, who had spent twenty years advising pregnant women to avoid local fish despite watching her community's traditional diets erode.

She wrote:

"We revised our guidance this year.

Your work is why.

No press release.

No headline.

Just a correction."

Another from a nutritionist in Hawaii:

"We were wrong about swordfish.

We should have looked at enzyme sufficiency.

I tell my students your model is what replaced the fear."

Another from a pediatric neurologist in Ireland:

"I didn't believe your early papers.

I apologize.

We're changing our counseling protocols."

These letters were never framed.

They were not shown to colleagues.

They were folded quietly into a drawer, each one a small, unceremonious confirmation that clarity was spreading in the only way clarity ever truly spreads:

one practitioner at a time.

Then came a letter that was different.

It was handwritten — unusual in any era, but especially in this one. The paper was thick. The handwriting precise. The address from a small coastal town where fishing traditions predated electricity.

He opened it slowly.

"Dr. Ralston,

I am not a scientist.

I am a mother.

For my first pregnancy I avoided fish.

For my second, once the guidance changed, I added it back.

The difference in my children is not subtle.

Thank you for correcting the story before it was too late for my daughter."

He sat still for a long time.

There had been conferences.

Symposiums.

Policy shifts.

Curricular revisions.

Textbook updates.

Institutional recalibrations.

But this letter —

this quiet, unadorned letter —

carried the truth of why the work began in the first place.

It wasn't about winning debates.

It wasn't about proving anything.

It wasn't about being right.

It was about giving one child —

and then another —

the neurological protection that comes only from a nutrient that had been hidden beneath a generation of fear.

He set the letter on his desk with reverence, not sentimentality.

Then he walked outside.

The river looked different today.

Not metaphorical.

Not symbolic.

Not a mirror.

Not a record.

Not continuation.

Today, the river looked like inheritance — the passage of something essential from one body to another, not through force, not through persuasion, but through the simple act of flowing.

The water was glassy near the banks, but faster in the center, a steady pulse cutting through the cold air. The clouds reflected across it in broken silver patterns that shifted with every gust of wind.

He leaned on the railing.

It occurred to him, in that moment, that the river had been teaching the model all along:

- that a system is only harmed when it is deprived of what sustains it,
- that the danger is not always the contaminant,
- that the true risk is insufficiency,
- that balance is stronger than avoidance,
- that movement is more protective than stagnation,
- that clarity arrives slowly, honestly, inevitably.

He closed his eyes.

He did not feel the weight of the past.

He felt the forward pull of everything that had finally begun to align.

The science was correct.

The world was adjusting.

The next generation was already standing on the stronger foundation.

And the river —

the river carried the continuity,

the correction,

the inheritance,

the future.

He breathed in slowly, the cold air sharpening his thoughts into something almost luminous.

He opened his eyes.

The work moved on.

There were evenings on campus when the buildings seemed to exhale — long, slow, architectural breaths that released the tension of decades. Tonight was one of those evenings. The sky was a soft charcoal blue, drained of color but rich with depth. A faint mist hovered near the streetlights, catching the light in thin halos.

Nick walked along the path that curved behind the science building, past the row of maples that had dropped the last of their leaves. The pavement was damp, carrying the scent of cold soil and limestone. He had no destination. His steps were unhurried, guided less by intention than by a quiet instinct to be near the spaces that had held his work through its long, uneven maturation.

He reached the courtyard behind the old research wing — a square of concrete framed by austere brick walls and a single bench worn smooth by winters. This was where he used to sit while waiting for lab results, eating cold lunches between experiments, occasionally wondering whether the model he carried would ever find its way into the world that resisted it.

He stepped into the center of the courtyard.

The lights from the building cast angled beams across the ground. The air felt heavier here — the kind of heaviness that comes not from pressure but from accumulation, like sediment settling slowly at the bottom of a riverbed.

For once, he wasn't thinking about data.

Or advisory language.

Or enzyme pathways.

Or policy drafts.

Or the global consensus that had taken shape around him.

He was thinking about time.

Not the passing of it, but the shaping of it.

There is a difference.

Time, in science, is rarely linear.

It bends.

It loops.

It stalls.

It accelerates.

It doubles back on itself.

Sometimes it collapses decades into a single moment.

Tonight felt like one of those collapses.

He could feel the twenty-five-year span contracting — the early doubts, the tentative findings, the external resistance, the internal certainty, the lonely conference talks, the overlooked diagrams, the cautious allies, the incremental studies, the slow, steady shift in global thought.

All of it settling into a single, quiet point in the courtyard.

He sat on the bench.

The stone was cold through his coat.

He let his hands rest on his knees, open, as though he were holding the air itself. The silence here was different from the silence by the river. The river's silence was movement; the courtyard's silence was memory.

He felt something he hadn't felt in years:

stillness.

Not the stillness of exhaustion.

Not the stillness of defeat.

But the stillness of recognition — the realization that the work had reached an altitude where it no longer relied on him to stay aloft.

It was flying on its own.

He wasn't stepping away.

He wasn't finishing.

He wasn't concluding.

He was witnessing.

Witnessing the rarest moment in a scientific life — the moment where your work becomes the environment in which others operate.

He leaned back slightly, letting the cool air settle against his collar.

He thought of the letters.

The global studies.

The curriculum changes.

The coastal mothers.

The researchers aligning their designs.

The clinicians rewriting their protocols.

The institutions softening their language.

The next generation learning the corrected model first.

He thought of all the people he would never meet who would nonetheless live in the world his work had helped to adjust.

And then he thought of the simplest truth:

The brain of a child —

a single, developing, unassuming brain —

would now grow with the nutrients it needed

because the science had finally been allowed

to become itself.

He closed his eyes.

There was no triumph in him.

No celebration.

No fatigue.

Only continuity — the long, quiet current of clarity moving through a world that was, at last, ready to accept it.

He stood slowly and walked out of the courtyard.

The river awaited him somewhere in the distance — steady, calm, patient — but tonight he did not need to see it.

He carried its movement within him.

There were mornings when the world felt like it had shifted by a single, imperceptible degree — a shift so slight that no headline would ever announce it, no institution would formally acknowledge it, yet anyone who had spent a lifetime watching patterns could feel the axis realign beneath their feet.

This was one of those mornings.

Nick woke early, not out of urgency but out of an old habit formed during the years when clarity had to be guarded, defended, explained, and sometimes carried alone. He brewed coffee in the quiet kitchen, listening to the faint mechanical hum of the university's heating system outside his window. He stood there for a moment, hands wrapped around the warm ceramic mug, absorbing a silence that felt unusually complete.

Something had ended.

Something had begun.

And both had happened quietly.

He walked to campus before the sun fully rose.

The sky was a pale, whispered blue. Frost clung to the edges of the sidewalks, thin enough to dissolve with the first touch of light. A few students hurried by, bundled in coats, carrying notebooks and half-formed ambitions.

He passed the library — lights still on from the night students who refused to surrender their final weeks of the semester. He passed the chemistry building, where someone had left a lamp glowing over a workstation. He passed the large auditorium where he had once given a guest lecture no one understood at the time, except for a single student who emailed him years later to say, "I think I get it now."

And then he reached the building that had been the center of his journey.

He didn't enter.

There was no need.

He stood on the steps, watching the slow drift of morning light across the windows.

This was the building where he had presented the early findings — the diagrams, the enzyme interactions, the balance model — and watched colleagues tilt their heads as though he were offering them a shape they had no category for.

This was where the resistance had lived.

Where the questions had sharpened.

Where the old model had defended itself out of habit, not accuracy.

Where the shift had begun in whispers long before it appeared in print.

He placed a hand on the railing, the cold metal grounding him.

Then he turned away from the entrance and walked toward the small footbridge that crossed into the older part of campus — the part students rarely visited unless they were lost or nostalgic.

Halfway across the bridge, he stopped.

Below him, a thin tributary split off from the main river — narrower, younger, but moving with the same direction and purpose, as though it carried a quiet memory of the larger current.

He watched it.

A tributary is not an imitation.

It is not a branch.

It is not a fragment.

A tributary is a continuation.

The main current had done its work.

Now the smaller bodies of water carried the motion forward — subtly, steadily, without the burden of origins.

He understood the metaphor instantly.

His work had become the main current.

Its continuation was now carried by others:

the young researcher in Southeast Asia,

the clinician in Ireland,

the doctoral student in Chile,

the public health nurse in Alaska,

the nutritionists,

the policy groups,

the new textbooks,

the updated curricula,

the quiet administrative drafts,

the letters,

the corrections,

the generational inheritance.

They were all tributaries now.

His contribution had moved into them.

Not his name.

Not his reputation.

Not his story.

The truth itself.

That was what mattered.

He leaned on the railing and watched the smaller stream merge back into the main river a few yards downstream.

Not in conflict.

Not in turbulence.

In harmony.

A merging so natural it barely disturbed the surface.

He stayed there for a long moment, feeling the strange, luminous clarity of a life's work entering its final, most elegant stage: not conclusion, not retirement, but diffusion.

The diffusion of truth into a world that was now prepared to hold it.

He stepped back from the railing, the cold morning air brushing lightly against his face.

There would still be conferences.

Still be questions.

Still be refinements.

Still be younger minds pushing the model further than he had imagined.

But the burden of correction — that long, heavy weight — had finally lifted.

He turned toward the east, where the sun was beginning to rise over the flat, open land.

The light spread slowly, evenly, without drama.

Exactly as it should.

There were afternoons when the world inside a laboratory felt distinctly different from the world outside it — as though time obeyed a separate physics behind those doors. This afternoon carried that feeling. The hallways were quiet, but the labs hummed faintly, alive with the low electrical pulse of centrifuges, incubators, and old refrigerators that never stopped working, even after the theories they once supported had been left behind.

Nick walked through the corridor with unhurried steps.

This building had once been the battlefield.

The old paradigm had lived here — in grant proposals, in whiteboard debates, in faculty lounges where people spoke in lowered voices, cautious not to appear too aligned with an idea that seemed, at first, too elegant to be believed.

But today, the atmosphere was simply... normal.

Students moved between rooms carrying pipettes and lab notebooks. A doctoral candidate was explaining her study design to an advisor in fluent biochemical shorthand. Two undergraduates were taping new printouts onto a poster board for an upcoming conference.

He could hear the soft click of keyboards, the whir of an orbital shaker, the rhythmic tap of someone pipetting samples in careful cadence.

What struck him was not the activity.

It was the absence of tension.

Once, this building had been the architecture of resistance.

Now, it had become the architecture of continuance.

He reached the end of the hall and stepped into one of the small teaching labs — the kind where foundational concepts are introduced before they ever reach a research setting.

A younger professor stood at the bench, setting up glassware for an afternoon demonstration. She looked up when she saw him.

"Oh — Dr. Ralston," she said, smiling. "Perfect timing. I'm about to teach the enzyme binding sequence. We're using your interaction model for the demonstration."

He nodded with quiet acknowledgment.

She did not say it like a compliment.

She said it like a fact.

She motioned to the whiteboard.

There, written in clean, precise handwriting, were the steps of the model — the cascade of biochemical dependencies he had spent years trying to articulate:

Selenium-binding priority

Enzyme activation hierarchy

Disruption thresholds

Mercury-binding competition

Balance-based vulnerability curves

He remembered writing these very same steps on far messier whiteboards two decades earlier, back when they elicited confusion, skepticism, or silence.

Now they were instructions.

Teaching tools.

Structured knowledge.

He asked, "Do the students grasp it easily?"

She laughed softly. "It's intuitive to them. I think the old model confuses them more."

He let that settle in.

The model that had once seemed unthinkably counterintuitive was now the simple one.

She lifted a pipette and began arranging small labeled vials of solutions along the bench.

"We run the enzyme interaction simulation," she explained, "and they can see how selenium saturation changes the entire vulnerability pattern. It makes the theory real for them."

Real.

He watched her work for a moment — the clarity in her movements, the certainty of someone building on a foundation she did not have to question.

Then she paused.

"By the way," she said, almost casually, "our graduate seminar is meeting next month. They're doing a session on the history of the paradigm shift. Would you like to attend? You wouldn't need to speak. Just... be there."

He smiled faintly.

A quiet smile, the kind that belongs to someone who recognizes an invitation not to be honored, but to be witnessed.

"I'll think about it," he said.

She nodded, turning back to her preparations.

He stepped out of the lab and into the hallway.

Outside, the light had changed again — afternoon sun giving way to the cooler tones of early evening. Shadows stretched long across the pavement as students headed toward the dining hall, the library, the river.

He walked that familiar path once more.

Not out of routine.

Out of recognition.

When he reached the riverbank, he paused.

Today, the river was not metaphor, not mirror, not continuation, not inheritance.

Today, the river was equilibrium — a quiet, perfect balancing of forces:

movement and stillness,

light and shadow,

depth and surface,

origin and arrival.

The water glided forward as though guided by an unseen symmetry, its center current dark and decisive, its edges soft and reflective.

He felt the symmetry inside himself.

For the first time in decades, the clarity he had carried did not feel like something pushing outward.

It felt like something returning inward.

The world had met the truth.

The field had aligned.

The next generation would carry the work further than he ever could.

He rested his hands on the railing.

There were no more battles to fight.

No more paradigms to defend.

No more misconceptions to unravel.

Only balance now.

The same balance he had been teaching for twenty-five years.

The same balance the river had always demonstrated without trying.

The same balance that would protect generations of children whose mothers would never know his name.

The water flowed on.

Balanced.

Precise.

Unhurried.

He let the quiet settle.

There were seasons in a scientist's life when the world no longer asked for explanation — only presence. This was one of those seasons. The semester was drawing to a close. Students were preparing for finals. Offices were cluttered with half-graded assignments and stacks of journal articles destined to be forgotten by spring. And yet the campus carried a quiet order, as though everything were aligning into its proper place before the year exhaled.

Nick walked through the long glass corridor that connected the research buildings. Late afternoon light angled through the windows, casting a warm, honey-colored glow across the polished floor. Dust motes drifted lazily in the beams of sun, illuminated for a moment before disappearing back into the air.

He reached the far end of the corridor and paused.

On the wall beside him was a digital screen that cycled through university announcements — guest lectures, faculty achievements, upcoming events. Most of it was routine: a seminar on renewable fuels, a visiting scholar in behavioral economics, a faculty recital from the music department.

Then a slide appeared that made him still.

It read:

"Maternal Health Workshop:

Updated Nutritional Frameworks and Clinical Applications."

Below it, in smaller text:

Featuring research from our faculty on selenium-dependent enzyme systems and fetal neurodevelopment.

No name.

No attribution.

Just the model.

He watched the slide loop back into rotation.

There was no thrill.

No ache.

Just a quiet sense of alignment — the satisfaction of seeing the truth installed inside the system it once strained to enter.

He continued down the hallway.

At the end of the corridor was a small, little-used seminar room. The door was ajar. Inside, a group of graduate students sat in a loose circle, notebooks open, laptops resting on crossed legs. They were in discussion — animated but orderly, the way serious students speak when they know the shape of an idea but not yet its depth.

He lingered at the door, unseen.

One student was speaking.

"Look, the reason the old model persisted so long isn't because it was right. It's because fear scales faster than nuance. And nuance takes a generation to reconstruct."

Another nodded. "That's why the interaction model matters — it shifts the entire premise. It says the vulnerability isn't the contaminant. It's the absence of the protective nutrient. Once you understand that, the whole picture clarifies."

A third added, "I can't imagine going back to the old warnings. They don't even make biochemical sense."

The conversation moved on — branching, deepening, refining. They cited studies he recognized, concepts he had introduced to the literature, phrases he had spent months trying to get exactly right. But they weren't quoting him. They were using the ideas as their own intellectual tools — the highest form of adoption.

He stepped quietly away from the door.

There was something profoundly humbling about hearing young minds debate a model that had once needed defending. They weren't guarding it. They weren't revering it. They were working with it, the way scientists work with oxygen or gravity — foundational truths that need no preface.

He left the seminar room behind.

Outside, the wind had picked up. The sky had shifted again — streaks of pale lavender against a field of deepening blue. The air smelled of distant snow, though none had fallen yet. He buttoned his coat and walked toward the river.

As he approached, he heard it before he saw it — a low, steady rush, the kind of sound that creates its own calm. When he reached the railing, he paused.

The river today was not metaphor, not record, not inheritance, not equilibrium.

Today, the river was permanence.

Not as a static thing — permanence rarely is — but as a sustained movement that endures regardless of season, weather, or witness.

The water flowed with a quiet authority, shaped not by force but by its own unbroken continuity. The surface shimmered with the fading light, scattering reflections into thin ribbons that dissolved as soon as they formed.

He rested his hands on the cold rail.

This was the stage of a scientific life no one teaches you to anticipate — the moment when the idea you carried ceases to be a burden, ceases to be a fight, ceases even to be "your work," and becomes simply the way the world now understands itself.

Not because you insisted.

Not because you persuaded.

But because the truth, once made visible, becomes the only model that makes sense.

He watched the river.

He felt no desire to control the narrative now, no need to ensure it would be remembered correctly. The model had entered its permanent form — installed in curricula, adopted in protocols, woven into research design, assumed by generations who would never know the fear it replaced.

He drew a slow breath.

If permanence has a feeling, it is this:

a quiet, steady release into continuity.

He stayed at the river's edge until the last light faded and the water turned the color of polished obsidian.

Then he stepped back from the railing, ready for whatever shape the next quiet movement would take.

There were winters on campus that arrived not with drama but with a kind of solemn inevitability — cold entering the air the way understanding eventually enters a field: quietly, steadily, without asking for permission. This winter had just begun. The first thin snow had fallen overnight, coating the sidewalks in a white, granular powder that crunched softly beneath each step.

Nick walked across the quad slowly, hands in his coat pockets, his breath rising in small, pale clouds. The buildings around him had taken on their winter personalities — darker windows, slower rhythms, a hush that came not from emptiness but from concentration. Winter is the season when thought deepens, when the world narrows to essential questions.

He welcomed it.

As he approached the research wing, he saw a notice posted on a bulletin board by the main entrance. The paper was crisp, freshly pinned. He stopped to read it.

"Call for Collaborative Proposals:

Fetal Neurodevelopment and Nutrient Interactions

In Partnership with International Centers for Maternal Health."

His eyes moved down the page.

"Priority will be given to studies evaluating nutrient competition models, including selenium-dependent enzyme protection in the context of environmental exposures."

He let the words settle.

Once, he had submitted proposals that included these very lines — and watched them go unfunded, dismissed as too speculative, too disruptive, too contrary to established messaging. And now, the institution was requesting them.

He continued reading.

"Research teams are encouraged to incorporate the updated framework in their proposals. Consultation with faculty familiar with the model is recommended."

He almost smiled at the understatement.

The model.

No name.

No citation.

No explanation.

Just the model — the one now native to the institution's bloodstream.

He turned from the notice and pushed open the door.

Inside, the building was warm, lit by a soft amber glow. He walked down the hallway, past the labs and offices that had once felt like trenches in a decades-long campaign. Today they felt like architecture — simple, orderly, no longer charged with tension.

As he passed one of the lecture rooms, he overheard a voice inside.

A guest lecturer.

He recognized the voice — a scientist from Europe, visiting for a short residency.

"...when evaluating vulnerability in the developing brain," she was saying, "the crucial variable is not mercury exposure in isolation, but the availability of selenium-dependent enzymes. The field now understands this. The public health messaging is beginning to follow."

A few students typed rapidly on laptops.

One raised a hand.

"So the older advisories were incomplete?"

The lecturer nodded, choosing her words carefully.

"Incomplete for their time, yes. But this is why science evolves. When new evidence becomes robust enough, guidance must shift. The interaction model gives us the clarity the older model lacked."

The student asked, "And that's now considered the consensus?"

"Yes," the lecturer said simply. "It is."

Consensus.

That word again — but here it carried a different weight.

It wasn't a citation.

It was a conclusion.

He stepped away from the door.

Outside, he continued toward the river on a narrow path that skirted the far edge of campus. The snow here was untouched, a thin white layer softening the landscape. His footsteps left a trail behind him, but the wind was already beginning to blur the edges.

When he reached the riverbank, he stopped.

Winter had begun its slow work on the water.

Thin sheets of forming ice clung to the edges.

The center current ran dark and smooth, unperturbed by the encroaching cold.

He leaned on the railing, watching.

The river today was not metaphor, not mirror, not continuation, not inheritance, not equilibrium, not permanence.

Today, the river was transition — the stage where two truths coexist without conflict:

the truth that has arrived,

and the truth that is still forming.

Ice and water.

Past and future.

Correction and expansion.

The field was in that same stage now.

The old warnings had not vanished entirely — pockets of outdated guidance still drifted through public health agencies, prenatal pamphlets, and the outskirts of international policy. But the new model had taken hold where it mattered:

in research design,

in curricula,

in clinical protocols,

in global discussions,

in the next generation's assumptions.

He rested his hands on the cold rail.

Transition is not the end.

Transition is the assurance that the end will not be needed.

He watched the slow pulse of the river, the water moving beneath the forming ice with steady resolve.

Something in him softened.

The work had reached its irreversible point.

The world would continue the correction now.

His job — the long, heavy part — was done.

He closed his eyes as the wind carried a few crystals of snow across his face.

When he opened them, the river was still moving.

Still dark.

Still sure.

Still true.

There were days when a scientist could feel the world narrowing to a single point, not because something was ending, but because something long dispersed was finally gathering itself into coherence. This was one of those days.

The morning sun rose weakly through a veil of thin winter cloud, casting a muted, diffused light over the campus. Snow clung to the edges of rooftops and window ledges. The air carried that brittle, crystalline stillness that makes sound travel farther and thought travel deeper.

Nick walked slowly across the quad, boots pressing into the thin crust of fresh snow. Students moved briskly around him, bundled in coats, their laughter rising in small bursts of warm breath. He watched them pass with a quiet recognition: they would never inherit the scientific confusion he spent twenty-five years dissolving. Their world was cleaner, lighter, sharper.

He approached the old administrative building—one of those structures whose hallways seemed to store institutional memory in the way old trees store rings. He entered, shaking the snow from his shoulders.

Inside, the hall was warm and dimly lit. A receptionist greeted him softly.

"They're expecting you upstairs."

Expecting him.

He climbed the staircase, its wooden steps creaking in a familiar rhythm. At the landing, he paused briefly before continuing to the conference room at the end of the hall.

Inside, a small group was seated around a long table. Administrators. Department chairs. A representative from public health. A faculty liaison. And at the far end, a young policy specialist who had flown in for this meeting.

They gestured for him to sit.

The chair began without ceremony.

"We're revising the university's external guidance on maternal nutrition," she said. "Not for publication yet. This is an internal draft."

A folder was passed to him.

He opened it.

He had seen many drafts in his career. But not like this.

The language was clear.

The science was accurate.

The framing was mature.

A paragraph caught his eye:

"The interaction model—now supported across multiple international studies—provides the most accurate framework for counseling on maternal seafood intake. Public messaging should shift from avoidance-based warnings to nutrient-sufficiency guidance."

He kept reading.

"Our institution adopts this model as standard, effective immediately. It reflects the consensus of the scientific community and aligns with global best practices."

Consensus.

Adopts.

Effective immediately.

He looked up slowly.

The chair spoke again, her tone measured but warm.

"We want to acknowledge the foundation your work provided. This transition would not be possible without it."

He said nothing for a moment.

For years, he had imagined what this acknowledgment might feel like—if it ever came at all. Vindication? Satisfaction? Relief?

But what he felt now was something far quieter:

alignment.

The kind of alignment that comes when a system finally matches the truth it resisted for decades.

Another administrator spoke.

“There’s also the matter of how we communicate this shift publicly. The messaging has to be careful, but honest.”

He nodded.

“Honesty is careful,” he said. “If you tell the public what we know now, not what we feared then, they will understand.”

The young policy specialist added, almost reverently:

“What you wrote twenty years ago… it’s becoming the global model. Countries are beginning to adapt it. Agencies, too. The change is real.”

He closed the folder gently, hands steady.

“Good,” he said. “That’s how it was always supposed to happen.”

They continued discussing logistics, timelines, advisory updates—but he no longer needed to guide the conversation. The work had its own voice now.

When the meeting ended, the chair walked with him to the door.

“One more thing,” she said softly. “You should know… this is only the beginning. Once the guidance shifts here, others will follow.”

He nodded, almost imperceptibly.

"Yes," he said. "They will."

Outside, the winter afternoon had softened into a faint, silver light. Snowflakes drifted lightly through the air, slow enough that each one seemed to navigate on its own terms.

He walked toward the river.

The path was quiet, coated in fresh snow. His footsteps left a simple pattern behind him, the prints already beginning to blur at the edges from the falling flakes.

When he reached the riverbank, he inhaled deeply.

Today, the river was not metaphor.

Not mirror.

Not continuation.

Not inheritance.

Not equilibrium.

Not permanence.

Not transition.

Today, the river was arrival.

The surface moved with a slow, luminous certainty, carrying the clarity of a truth that no longer needed advocacy. The forming ice hugged the edges but did not impede the current. A soft mist hovered above the water, catching what little light remained.

He leaned on the railing.

Arrival is not a moment.

It is a recognition.

A recognition that the truth has reached the place it was always meant to occupy,

that the field has absorbed what once felt unabsorbable,

that the resistance has dissolved into understanding,

that the world has caught up to the science.

He exhaled.

The river flowed on.

Not toward conclusion—

toward continuity.

He watched it until the light dimmed completely.

There were late-winter evenings when the world felt as though it were holding something in reserve — not withholding, not concealing, but simply waiting for the right moment to let the final shape of a season emerge. This was one of those evenings.

The sky had taken on the muted indigo of a day beginning its quiet retreat. A thin glaze of frost coated the pavement, making each step sound like a faint, crystalline whisper. The campus buildings glowed softly from within, their windows illuminated like small squares of persistence against the early dark.

A final movement was approaching.

Not announced.

Not declared.

But unmistakable.

Nick walked along the northern path, the one that curved behind the older buildings where the university kept its archives and its long-unused lecture halls. He preferred this route for reasons he never articulated — perhaps because this part of campus carried the weight of its own history without embarrassment. It reminded him that institutions evolve not by forgetting their past, but by absorbing it.

He stopped at a side entrance: a door he had passed thousands of times but rarely used. Something drew him to it now.

Inside was a narrow hallway lined with framed photographs — black-and-white portraits of faculty from decades earlier, their expressions austere, their attire formal, their lives entirely contained within the silent spaces between shutter clicks. Most were unknown to him. A few he recognized.

He walked slowly, reading the small brass nameplates beneath each frame.

Here was a chemist whose work had been rejected for years before becoming foundational.

Here was a nutritionist who pushed for a new model of deficiency long before anyone believed her.

Here was a physiologist who rewrote an entire field through a single insight no one understood at the time.

Here were the faces of those who had carried truths before the world knew what to do with them.

He reached the end of the hallway.

A lone frame hung on the wall.

Empty.

The brass nameplate beneath it read only:

“Reserved for Emerging Contributions.”

He stared at the empty frame for a long time.

Not because he imagined his own portrait hanging there — he didn’t. He had never sought that kind of legacy. The emptiness spoke to something else:

that every field carries its own expectancy,

its own invitation to clarity,

its own space for the work that must come next.

He stepped back from the frame.

The emptiness was not waiting for him.

It was waiting for the generation he had helped orient.

He left the hallway quietly.

Outside, the light had fallen into that rare winter luminance where everything — buildings, trees, snow, sky — seemed cut from a single sheet of pale steel. The river was visible from this vantage point, a dark, unwavering line through the frozen landscape.

He moved toward it.

This time, the path was unfamiliar — not one he normally took. It veered behind the engineering building, descended a small incline, and led to a lower overlook that most people ignored, preferring the broader view from the main bridge.

He reached the railing.

The river below was a study in contradictions — half-ice, half-water, shifting subtly between stillness and motion. Along the edges, delicate ice patterns formed and reformed in slow fractal spirals. In the center, the water cut through like a vein of living darkness.

Tonight, the river was threshold —

the moment between what has been corrected

and what will continue beyond correction.

A threshold is not a beginning.

Nor is it an ending.

It is the point at which both coexist.

He rested both hands on the railing, letting the cold seep into his palms.

He thought of the generations ahead — the scientists who would refine the model, expand it, challenge it, elevate it, transform it into iterations he could never predict. He thought of the clinicians who would adopt it, not out of revolution, but out of routine. He thought of the mothers whose decisions would be shaped by corrected guidance rather than inherited fear. He thought of the children whose brains would grow under the protection of nutrients once misunderstood.

He closed his eyes.

For the first time in his life, he felt the split-second clarity that arrives only when a lifetime of work aligns into a single, undeniable truth:

It was never about being right.

It was about leaving the world with fewer ways to be wrong.

The cold wind brushed past him, carrying with it the faint scent of winter's slow retreat.

He opened his eyes again.

The threshold lay before him — the place where his work ended and its continuity began.

The river moved with steady precision, cutting forward through ice that could not hold it.

He remained there until the darkness folded completely around the landscape, the river becoming a long, quiet shadow moving through the night.

When he finally stepped back from the railing, he did so with the understanding that a final movement was still ahead — not as conclusion, but as the last, necessary settling of the truth into its final shape.

There were final movements in a long scientific life that did not feel like endings at all, but like clarifications — the last, subtle adjustments that allow the whole structure to stand without strain. They come not with applause, not with ceremony, but with an internal quiet that feels earned rather than granted.

This was one of those movements.

A gentle snow had begun falling in the early hours, thin flakes drifting down with the unhurried confidence of a season that knew exactly what it was doing. The campus was muted, softened, dressed in a pale layer of newness that made every footstep sound deliberate.

Nick crossed the quad slowly.

He was not on his way to a meeting.

Not to a lecture.

Not even to a lab.

He was walking toward a place he had avoided for years:

the archive.

The university archive — that subterranean repository where the institution kept what it could not yet categorize. Shelved manuscripts. Unfinished dissertations. Obscure conference proceedings. Failed grant proposals. Letters from donors long forgotten. Boxes of research materials waiting for their context to arrive.

The archive was the university's memory of what the world wasn't ready for at the time it was created.

He descended the narrow staircase, the air growing cooler with each step. At the bottom, a librarian greeted him with a knowing nod.

"You're here to see the early files," she said, as though this moment had been anticipated.

He nodded.

She led him down a hallway of metal shelves and dim lights until they reached a row marked Early 2000s—Biochemistry & Nutrition.

She pulled out a box labeled only with a date he remembered all too well.

She set it on the table and left him alone with it.

He opened the lid slowly.

Inside were the early documents he had long forgotten:

- The first draft of the enzyme-interaction hypothesis.
- Notes from the dive expedition that changed his trajectory.
- Early data tables with handwritten corrections in the margins.
- A letter he had written to a federal agency, never answered.
- Reviewer comments from a journal rejecting his manuscript.
- A printed email from a colleague warning him not to “push the model too far.”
- Conference slides with diagrams no one understood at the time.
- A folded note from a graduate student thanking him for explaining it twice that day.

He lifted each piece gently, placing them in a loose chronological order on the table.

There, spread before him, was the entire origin story — the work as it existed before it had language, before it had acceptance, before it had shape.

He sat down.

One by one, he reread the documents.

Not with nostalgia.

Not with regret.

With recognition.

These were not failures.

These were the starting points.

The places where clarity began before the world had the tools to receive it.

He touched the corner of an early diagram — the enzyme hierarchy sketched with a dull pencil on printer paper — and realized with a jolt of quiet certainty:

This diagram, this fragile, tentative thing,

is now the foundation of an entire field.

He leaned back slowly in the chair.

The archive was never about preservation.

It was about waiting.

Waiting for the moment when the early truth could be reabsorbed into the final one.

He gathered the papers, placed them back in the box, and closed the lid.

He did not feel the need to keep any of it.

He did not need the origin story validated.

It had done its work.

He stood, thanked the librarian, and stepped back into the winter light.

Outside, the snow had stopped. The sky was a luminous, pale gray — one of those winter skies that looks less like atmosphere and more like a sheet of light suspended above the earth.

He walked toward the river with measured steps.

When he reached the overlook, he stopped.

Today, the river was resolution —

not conclusion,

not finality,

but the quiet, steady settling of everything into its rightful place.

The ice near the banks had thickened.

The central channel still moved, dark and certain.

The line between ice and water had softened into a gradient — no clear boundary, no conflict, only transition becoming shape.

He rested his hands on the railing.

The work had entered its final movement not because it had ended, but because it no longer needed him to sustain it.

Resolution is not the cessation of effort.

Resolution is the moment the effort becomes self-sustaining.

He watched a thin crack expand across the ice near the far bank — silent, natural, inevitable. It did not threaten the structure. It completed it.

He breathed out slowly, watching his breath dissolve into the air.

The river flowed.

The ice held.

The winter settled around him.

The world, at last, had synchronized with the truth.

He stood there a long time, listening to the near-silent hum of a river in winter — the sound of resolution made visible.

There were endings in a scientist's life that did not declare themselves. They did not rise with crescendo or fall with collapse. They arrived the way clarity always does: quietly, exactly when the world is prepared to receive it. And in this final movement, everything that had unfolded over decades — the resistance, the recalibration, the alignment, the inheritance — gathered into a single, unmistakable point of recognition.

The day was cold, but not severe.

A light snow drifted in the air, almost hesitant.

The sun hovered behind a veil of winter cloud, softening the landscape to the color of pale ash.

Nick walked slowly along the river path.

He did not need to go to the lab.

He did not need to meet with students.

He did not need to review drafts or revise guidance.

All of those things would continue without him.

He walked because he wanted to see the shape of the river on the day the work reached completion — not the completion of the science itself, which would live far beyond him, but the completion of his role within it.

He reached the overlook and leaned on the familiar railing.

The river was half-ice, half-water — a long, dark vein moving through a frozen landscape with a certainty that no season could erase. Ice patterns glistened along the edges: fractal spirals, delicate fans, small crystalline plates overlapping with quiet intention.

The water at the center moved steadily, its motion barely perceptible unless one watched closely.

It was the perfect form of resolution.

He stood there, letting the cold air settle around him.

The river he had visited through every stage of this journey had taken on a new form today — not metaphor, not memory, not mirror, not transition, not permanence, not threshold.

Today, the river was continuance.

A pure, unbroken line between what his life had carried

and what the world would now carry alone.

He closed his eyes.

He thought of the early days — the empty seminar rooms, the skeptical colleagues, the hesitant funding bodies, the endless recalculations. He thought of the years when clarity felt like an upstream motion against the weight of institutions. He thought of the mothers who feared the wrong thing. He thought of the children who deserved a truer model. He thought of the scientists who slowly aligned, the young researchers who took the model into their own hands, the global voices who absorbed the truth without drama.

He thought of the tributaries.

He thought of the archive.

He thought of the quiet shift in the seminar rooms, the updated curricula, the new textbooks, the corrected guidance, the letters from distant shorelines.

He thought of how strange it was that the world had changed without announcing that it was changing.

And then he opened his eyes.

A single snowflake landed on the railing — fragile, crystalline, perfect. It melted within seconds, absorbed into the cold metal. It was a small thing. But it reminded him that everything, eventually, returns to the environment that sustains it.

Truth is no different.

It returns to the world, not to the person who carried it.

He drew a slow, steady breath.

It was time.

Not to leave.

Not to conclude.

But to release.

He placed both hands on the railing and spoke softly into the cold air — not to be heard, but to acknowledge the moment:

"It's yours now."

He meant the work.

He meant the truth.

He meant the future.

The river moved beneath him, dark and certain, as though receiving the words into its current.

He stepped back one pace from the railing.

The landscape around him was still, but not static.

The world had begun to move in alignment with something he had once carried alone.

This was the closing cadence —

the quiet, final settling of a story whose purpose had always been larger than its author.

He turned from the river and walked slowly up the path, the snow crunching softly beneath his boots, the cold air filling with the faint promise of a coming season.

Behind him, the river continued its motion, unbroken.

Ahead of him, the world opened calmly.

And the work, finally, beautifully, irreversibly, continued without him.

POSTSCRIPT

There are scientific journeys that resolve themselves in publications, policy changes, or accolades. And then there are journeys like this one—where the resolution is quieter, more diffused, woven into the daily decisions of people who may never know the origin of the clarity they now inherit. The work reflected in these pages does not rest on conclusion, because it was never built on argument. It was built on observation, patience, and the refusal to abandon accuracy in a world that often rewards urgency instead.

In many ways, this long essay is not an ending but a continuation. The model will be refined, expanded, challenged, and defended by those who come after. Guidance will keep shifting toward the truth that took decades to articulate. The developing brain will benefit from a truer understanding of what nourishes it. And the scientist who carried the model through the long winters of resistance has quietly stepped into the natural anonymity of a field that now moves in alignment with the work he began.

The river through which this narrative has flowed will continue its course long after these pages close. Its current now moves with the persistence of corrected knowledge, carrying the next generation into a world that has fewer ways to be misled. In this, there is a certain peace. Not triumph. Not vindication. Simply the satisfaction of knowing that the truth has finally synchronized with the world that needed it.

ABOUT THE AUTHOR

Joe Cozart is the founder of GMJoe™ Consulting, where clarity, structural narrative, and sovereign thinking define the core of his work. He is recognized for a literary approach that blends elegant recursion with strategic insight, producing long-form essays that explore the quiet architecture of systems, institutions, and the individuals who shape them. His body of work spans aerospace, scientific research, economic ecosystems, and high-society essays, all unified by a singular conviction: that clarity is sovereignty.

His published canon includes major works such as The Night Manager, The Velvet Edge, The Grand Forks Complex, The Enigma Cycle, and the Continuum series. His writing has become known for its disciplined tone, recursive elegance, and the subtle intelligence that invites readers into deeper layers of understanding without ever announcing the mechanism. Whether writing on clandestine aerospace doctrine, university research landscapes, or the quiet shifts in global science, he approaches each subject with reverence for accuracy and an ear tuned to the deeper music beneath the observable world.

He lives and works in Grand Forks, North Dakota, drawing insight from the region's unique convergence of scientific research, defense infrastructure, and northern quietude. His ongoing work continues to expand the interplay between literary craft and strategic clarity, establishing a body of writing that serves both as narrative and as record.

GMJoe™ is a trademark of Joe Cozart. © 2025 All rights reserved.

Made in the USA
Monee, IL
12 November 2026

a0f8d72b-f852-47b9-a8d3-db7ebd3a0997R01